RUN YOUR FIRST MARATHON

ALSO BY GRETE WAITZ

On the Run (with Gloria Averbuch)
Opp! Fra 0 til 100 paa 10 (*Up! From 0 to 100 in 10 Weeks*)
Stress ned kom i form (*Conquer Stress*)
(with Willi Railo and Sigmund Stromme)
World Class (with Gloria Averbuch)

ALSO BY GLORIA AVERBUCH

A Turn for Lucas
Goal! (with Ashley Michael Hammond)
It's Not About the Bra (with Brandi Chastain)
Joan Samuelson's Running for Women (with Joan Benoit Samuelson)
The New York City Marathon Cookbook (with Nancy Clark)
New York Road Runners Complete Book of Running & Fitness, Fourth Edition
New York Road Runners Running & Fitness Log 2007
On the Run (with Grete Waitz)
The Vision of a Champion (with Anson Dorrance)
The Woman Runner
World Class (with Grete Waitz)

RUN YOUR FIRST MARATHON

Everything You Need to Know to Make It to the Finish Line

Grete Waitz
and Gloria Averbuch

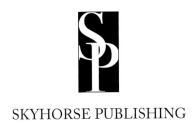

SKYHORSE PUBLISHING

www.skyhorsepublishing.com

ISBN-10: 1-60239-120-3
ISBN-13: 978-1-60239-120-8

This book is designed to provide you with guidance about your marathon, exercise, and fitness program. Although every effort has been made to provide the most careful and up-to-date advice, including in the medical field, this book is not intended as a substitute for any treatment or advice offered by a medical professional. You should seek medical approval before undertaking any exercise program.

Photos courtesy of New York Road Runners.

Stretching and strengthening photos of Grete Waitz by Vebjorn Rogne, courtesy of Schibsted ASA.

Library of Congress Control Number: 2007937054

10 9 8 7 6 5 4 3 2 1

Printed in the United States of America

CONTENTS

For my family, through thick and thin; my husband, Jack, who has seen me through all the miles—on the road and in life; and to my brothers, Jan and Arild.

— *G.W.*

To my daughters, Yael and Shira, the most inspiring athletes I know.

— *G.A.*

INTRODUCTION

Almost thirty years ago, I lined up for my first marathon. Little did I know then how much that event would change my life.

This is a sentence that can also be uttered by the multitudes of those who have done what I have—and what you will do: run your first 26.2-mile race.

I can't promise you a life-altering experience, just as I can't predict your race time. But one thing of which I feel certain: While not all of us can climb Mt. Everest, we can complete a marathon. I understand what that means, and what it takes. So does my co-author, Gloria.

I am asked all the time by aspiring marathoners if I can help them to realize their dream, whether they are strangers, acquaintances, friends, or family. Most of them aren't even runners. They request a training program, or even just some words of advice or encouragement. Having had a full and wonderful career, made possible by the magic of the 26.2-mile race, I always give the same answer. Yes!

I know what a great achievement it is to run a marathon, and I want to share that with you. I respect and understand what it takes to go the distance, and I know I can take you there. I've provided novice marathoners with everything from basic outlines to detailed training programs and advice, and I've watched and shared the joy and success of so many of them over the years. Of all those I have been privileged to work with, every one of them said they were glad they took on the challenge.

My marathon career opened up a whole new world for me. And I have seen it do the same for so many of those whom I have trained, including Gloria. And so, she and I—both of us marathoners and authors who have written books and articles together for twenty years, but even more, have been close friends—have teamed up to do it again. This time, we have created a blueprint for all of you new to our sport. Like you, Gloria and I were once first-time marathoners, and what we gained in knowledge and understanding from running that race has remained and been strengthened. Now into our fifties, we are both still avid runners and exercisers. Like every veteran of the marathon, we reflect fondly on that first experience. What we share with you in this book has been constructed by years of participation and experimentation, and with the help of some of the best minds in our sport. We hope you will truly benefit from our collective wisdom.

May your road ahead be a smooth one, filled with the same sense of adventure and discovery that ours has been.

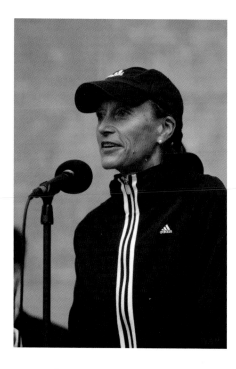

1

Why Run?

Once upon a time, I, too, was a first-time marathoner, although my experience was vastly different than what it is for runners today and, undoubtedly, what it will be for you. I ran my first marathon in 1978, in what you could call the "dark ages." The marathon fever that eventually broke out during the 1980s running-boom wasn't yet born. In those early days, few even knew what a marathon was (26.2 miles), let alone talked about the event. In fact, even those who ran the marathon on the national level were thought of as "strange." And that was among fellow runners!

Times have changed since then. Today, marathoning is increasing in popularity year by year. According to the latest statistics from Running USA's Road Running Information Center at www.runningusa.org, the estimated U.S. marathon finisher total for 2006 is 410,000. That's up from 395,000 in 2005. Mirroring a nationwide trend, about half the entrants, on average, in the half-dozen or so

Rock n' Roll marathon race series are first-timers—also true for nearly that many in the New York City Marathon, the largest marathon in the world.

Back in 1978, I was a twenty-five-year-old full-time schoolteacher who ran with my hair in pigtails. I had never been to the United States. I had absolutely no expectations of the marathon, except to use it as a way to get a trip to this country before I retired from running. I was a top track runner in Europe, but I was about to close that chapter of my life and, in so doing, complete my running career. The longest I had ever raced was 3,000 meters, but that didn't seem to matter. New York City Marathon race director Fred Lebow offered to bring me over to act as a rabbit (pacesetter). A rabbit is expected to drop out of a race, but to pull the race favorites to a good time before she does. He figured that I might only make it through the longest distance I had ever run to that point (twelve miles in training), but that at least I would do it quickly.

When I got to the starting line, I didn't even know where to stand. The New York City Marathon start on the Verrazano-Narrows Bridge was a virtual sea of people, an overwhelming sight for someone used to standing with a handful of runners on the track.

Obviously, I had no idea what it meant to run 26.2 miles. If you have not run the full marathon distance in training before (which very few runners have, and not many experts recommend doing), at some point you enter unknown territory. You go beyond anything you have ever done. Obviously, with my twelve-mile training background, I reached that point very soon.

As is true for so many novice marathoners, the race started off pretty well for me. I was certainly running at a far more comfortable pace than during a track race, with the added push of the spectators cheering us on. However, as the miles clicked by, I had no idea where I was or how far I had run, never having seen the course. I heard the mile split times, but I was mystified, since as a European, I was schooled in running by kilometers. I was too tired, and too drained, to try to convert the miles to a distance I could comprehend. Every time I turned a corner and saw a tree, I prayed it was Central Park, since I knew that was where the race finished. (Contrary to popular belief, and unfortunately for me that day, there are many parts of New York City with lots of trees.) I tried to take water at the aid stations, but since I wasn't used to drinking on the run, it just went all over my face and up my nose. There was no such thing as a sports drink along the way, not to mention energy gels—both inventions of the future.

Eventually, this new experience came to a conclusion, thank goodness. To everyone's surprise, including my own, I finished with a then world-record

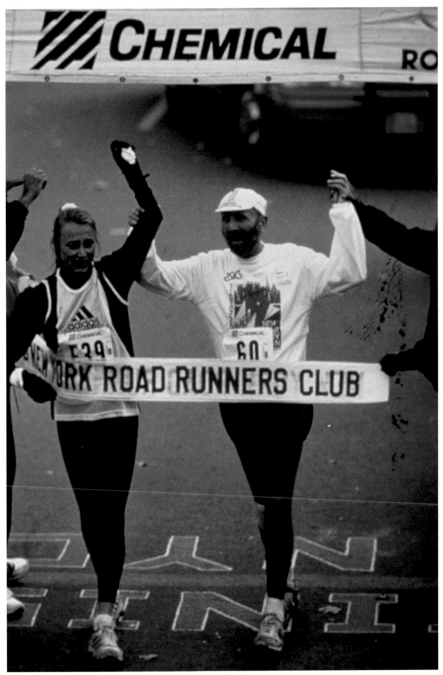

Finishing my most emotional marathon in 1992, with my friend, the late New York City Marathon race director Fred Lebow.

time (2:32:30). So unexpected was it for me to even cross the line, let alone win, that the announcer and the press didn't know who I was. "Who is number 1178?" (my running bib) could be heard circulating throughout the finish area. It remains the most famous line of my career. Make no mistake. I was able to run, and run well, because of my strong track background (and my willpower). But basically, I did it without a clue. The entire experience was a bizarre one.

I finished my first marathon not necessarily because I was well prepared, but for other reasons. Track running is a very demanding sport, so I did "speak the language." But even more, it is my personality type to finish what I start. I had never dropped out of a track or cross-country race, unless I was injured. I am a very organized, methodical, and disciplined person. Now, lest you think I've got it all together, I'll give you the real "bottom line" reason I kept going that day. I knew I had to finish, because if I dropped out, I had no idea where I was (a stranger in a strange city); I had no money and no clue how I would get back if I didn't continue to "follow the pack." However, the basic traits that got me through it will, as I will emphasize, work for you as well.

No matter who we are, at some point we are all first-time marathoners. All of us share that. That's the beauty of the race—Olympians and all-comers share the same event. We all set a goal for ourselves. We all work hard. We all seek to be surrounded by others who will encourage and support us. However, although you and I may share some things in common, in certain fundamental ways you will be so much better off in your first marathon than I was. Unlike me, you will face the race with excitement and some knowledge of what you can expect. You will not run in paper-thin shoes, like I did; you will instead benefit from a wide variety of supportive, shock-absorbing models. Unlike me, you will study the course and complete a series of training runs, scientifically designed to prepare you for the marathon experience. Unlike me, you will take advantage of all the nutritional and training breakthroughs that have so revolutionized the sport. And whether you complete the race only one time (as I swore to do the minute I crossed the finish line in 1978), or go on to duplicate your feat (which I did at least twice a year for the next decade), you will become part of the society of those who have conquered this modern day Everest.

Although I describe a somewhat sorry tale of my first marathon, the truth is that it opened up a whole new world for me. I began a second running career, which became the source of my greatest professional and personal satisfaction. Some of my reasons for running the marathon were the same as yours. The distance is a challenge. (Of course, winning it was an even bigger challenge.) Breaking the world record that first time—which I did three more times before the end of my career—especially motivated me. And while records can be broken, victories are forever. Although victory for me meant crossing the line first, you, too, will experience a personal victory. The marathon may inspire you to find strength and discipline you never knew you possessed; you may overcome sadness, fear, or doubt in order to run; you may want to prove that even in middle age, you're "not done yet." Whatever defines a "victory" motivates us all and makes the 26.2-mile journey worth the preparation that goes into it.

Aside from all the differences that separate us, the magic we share will be the same. Before I ran a marathon, I circled a track, sometimes with only a handful of spectators. And even a full stadium could not compare to what I

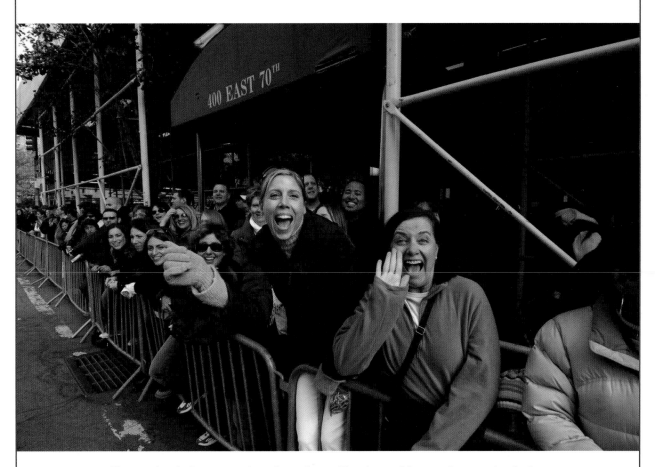

The marathon is the stage, and you the performer. The cheers of the crowd are your inspiration.

experienced in a big-city marathon. It is the entirety of the event, the whole package, which still makes me marvel. Even though it was tough getting to the finish line, I realized as soon as I crossed it that first time that the atmosphere of the marathon is something special. Depending on what race you run, you might be among hundreds or thousands of people on that starting line, sharing something unique and special. Perhaps there will be spectators cheering you along every mile of the route. In New York, the entire city gets into the Marathon.

The New York City Marathon receives over 70,000 applications and can only accept 35,000 runners. And those are just the people who decide to give applying to it a try, knowing it's up to the luck of the lottery to get in. My friend and New York City Marathon race director, the late Fred Lebow, was asked the question, "Why do so many people run the marathon?" all the time. He had an answer I like. He said that beyond the more obvious reasons, like getting in shape and social status, it's because we need to test ourselves, both physically and psychologically. "We can't sprout wings and fly. Most of us can't sing or dance, and we'll never perform on the stage," he said. But for a day, we can perform, often in front of millions of people. "It's like being on Broadway and getting a standing ovation!" was the way Fred put it. For a day, we can all be champions.

I've been asked over the years if I got more satisfaction from winning marathons than from winning races at other distances. Winning is always satisfying, but when you succeed in a marathon, it stays with you. It may be (or at least feel like) a piece of cake, or it may be tough going. You'll undoubtedly feel it in your legs for a while, but that passes. You will feel the sweetness of the achievement forever.

As a first-time marathoner in the twenty-first century, you will go down a completely different road than I did all those years ago. With the help of this book, you will have all the latest information and access to all the programs and gadgets. Enjoy your journey.

Now—let's get started!

WHAT CAN YOU EXPECT?

Obviously, every person is different. If you are completely new to sports and exercise, you'll start from scratch. You'll also have the prospect of a new adventure to spur your enthusiasm and excitement, in addition to a lot of relatively new benefits, such as a wealth of cutting-edge information and a tried-and-true training program. If you have had some athletic background, you have an advantage. To some degree, you probably already have a feel for physical training; maybe you are mentally competitive and more confident you can finish what you begin. However, be careful not to let past experience and what you did in your "younger days" overly influence you. The marathon has unique demands. I have known many runners, even world-class runners, who were humbled by it.

Whatever your level of experience, and perhaps alongside a sense of excitement, you will likely also experience an understandable apprehension. I coached Pittsburgh Steelers football legend Lynn Swann when he ran the marathon for the first time. He approached it as an athlete, but he had one feeling all rookies seem to share: he was nervous. Lynn was very much like the thousands of others I meet. Every year, I sign autographs at the race Expos for major marathons. If you multiply those I've met in these crowded Expos over the years, you'll have an idea of how many marathoners I encounter—up to half of whom are rookies. Almost every one of them expresses the same sense of doubt that Lynn did. They are anxious. They are afraid they will hurt. They doubt themselves. "I just hope I can make it to the finish line," they tell me. And if they do finish, they're afraid they will finish last.

I always give the autograph seekers the same advice I will give you: If you are healthy and uninjured when you get to the race; if you have done the "homework"—the proper training—including a number of long runs coupled with adequate recovery; if you eat and drink appropriately, and you pace yourself wisely, you're going to make it.

My sister-in-law Wenche is an average person. She is 52 and works full-time as a nurse. Although she is a health-minded gym-goer, she had never been a runner. This, despite the fact she is surrounded by her husband, brothers-in-law, and me, all of whom have run many marathons over many years. But she obviously had her eye on us all. For years it had been her dream to run one, too. "I don't know if I can make it," she confided in me. "Of course you can," I replied. Following the basic program I have published for the first time in this book, she completed the 2006 New York City Marathon, using a combination of jogging with walk breaks, in a very respectable time of 4:22.

One of the other people I trained to run his first marathon is a television comedian in Norway, who at the time was in his mid-forties. Unlike Wenche, he was not even into general fitness. He "got the bug" to run a marathon by completing a 5K; over time, and with an eye toward the full distance, he also did a half marathon. He was very nervous as the 26.2-mile race approached. He had nightmares and didn't sleep well. The night before the race, he had to get up in the middle of the night and take a shower, because his nightmares made him sweat so much. He was overweight when he started his training, but lost about twenty-five pounds during the course of his preparation. He was still heavy when he ran the marathon, but he clocked an impressive time of a little over four hours. It was a big personal victory for him. At the time he ran, twenty years ago, fewer people understood what it took to do a marathon. Needless to say, those he encountered were very impressed.

Most people are apprehensive because they have expectations, either from reading about the race or hearing other people's experiences. Then they try to imagine themselves going through it. In my case, I wasn't nervous the first time because I didn't know what to be nervous about. I had no idea what I was in for. No one expected anything from me, and I didn't expect anything from myself. In later marathons, when I had a public reputation and a personal goal, I was nervous every single time. Despite past success, I always asked myself, Why am I doing this? There was pressure from the outside, and I put pressure on myself. I was expected to win. But I knew then, and still believe, as the expression goes, that "If you're not nervous, it's time to hang up your shoes." Positive nervousness is what keeps you going. You need to know that apprehension is part of the challenge, and when you understand how it can work for you, you'll learn to appreciate it as part of the experience.

From the time you begin the training program until the moment you stand on the starting line, you may feel anxious. I don't think you can avoid being nervous. It gets the adrenaline going; it motivates you and helps you to perform. But it's important not to let anxiety take over, to spend too much energy focusing on the "big goal," which in the beginning is far off, or to focus on what you can't control. Take it one step at a time.

Apprehension takes a turn for the worse when it becomes fear. Even my first time, I was never really afraid. For one thing, having no clue what to expect, the old cliché turned out to be true: ignorance is bliss. But most importantly, as I will impress upon you over and over, I did the one thing that guaranteed I was going to make it: I went out slowly and ran conservatively, which gave me the security of knowing I was basically in control.

Unlike when I began running the marathon, these days everyone knows about the event. And they are impressed when you run one. Wenche's boss and her patients gave her a lot of support before she ran and even more hearty congratulations when she returned to work after the race. Of course, respect comes from finishing, and the fact that you gain physical fitness and health benefits from getting into shape for the race is a bonus. But there is also the dream. When you line up in New York, Chicago, or for the Rock 'n' Roll marathon in San Diego or Phoenix—all with bands and fans along the course and a lot of other runners (including first-timers) to keep you company—it's to have a complete experience. You may go the distance only once, but it is my sincere hope that you do it as a celebration.

GOALS AND MOTIVATION

Probably the most common reason that people take on the marathon is to get in shape. Everybody wants to be fit. Most of the people I've helped over the years have that as a goal. Some people undertake the marathon to celebrate an event—such as a major birthday. One woman I worked with got a fiftieth birthday present from her husband: an entry, including the trip, to the New York City Marathon. A lot of people do it to raise money for charity. I am proud that as a cancer survivor, I have personally been the focus of a charity. In the 2005 New York City Marathon, Fred's Team, comprised of 800 in that race, raised two million dollars for cancer research in my name, with the motto "Running for Grete Waitz."

Many people see the marathon as their personal Everest; they want to do it simply because "it's there." There's also a lot of wagering. People decide to do it on a whim, or a dare. Once, our neighbor asked me how fast I could run. I told him 2:24. It seemed logical to him he could go the distance in an extra hour. So we bet on it. In the end, he ran the London marathon in 4:40 and had so many blisters on his feet he literally had to travel back to Norway barefoot. I won a bottle of red wine.

If betting adds a little fun to your incentive, by all means risk the gamble. Right now, my brother Jan has a bet going with his son, Terje. Terje, once a fit little boy and young man, is now a thirty-five-year-old overweight guy whose only running these days is to chase his children's soccer ball. Jan is a fit sixty-two-year-old who runs New York every year. He has bet $30,000 that Terje cannot beat his father in the 2007 New York race (held on November 4). This spring, Terje, in fact, began his marathon training. I spoke with him in April and was somewhat encouraged to discover that he is already up to running continuously for ninety minutes. He cross trains by running three times a week and playing soccer twice a week. He's lost twenty pounds so far. I guess he's taking his bet with his father seriously. I, too, have a wild and long-standing bet with Jan: $50,000 says he will not break 3:30 (which he hasn't done in about a decade). That bet is his motivation, but I'm confident that my money is safe.

You can achieve your goal if you take the time to do the homework—that is, the training. To make sure you create an ideal incentive, choose a special marathon to run, such as one in a city you would like to visit, or a race you have heard of or dreamed about. Enter the event with friends or a running group to further motivate you. Choose a cause to run for, such as a charity, if that will inspire you. All of these factors will help get you out the door to train on dark or cold days.

Set this philosophy in stone: Your goal is to make it to the finish line. The clock is not your motivation; it's only there to make sure you stay on pace. Train your mind to not only accept this, but to also embrace it. It frees you from the stress of excessive ambition. Trust me, running for time in your first marathon can be your downfall, because even with race experience, achieving a goal time is extremely difficult. On the other hand, proper pacing should be your security blanket. You don't want to be without it. When I ran the first time, I had little idea about pacing. I didn't know if I was running 2:32 or 3:32. When rookies tell me they want to run to meet a goal time, I always question them: Do you know what pace that is? Have you done the training? Are you comfortable at that pace? I want to make sure their goal is realistic, because it is amazing how big a gap there often is between expectations and reality.

Make your marathon undertaking a positive experience. Vow to enjoy it from beginning to end, because you will work hard. But from your training through to race day, it should be satisfying work, not drudgery or stress. It's hard to train alone, so before you even lace up your shoes, find some friends or a running group or club. Get your friends, family, and coworkers involved by asking them to pledge to your charity, or have pre- or post-training meals or picnics together.

Don't think too much about the actual marathon in the early stages. Focus on short-term or intermediate goals, such as: "In three weeks, I'm doing a 10K; in twelve weeks, I'm running a half-marathon." Take a lesson from experienced runners, who always have the satisfaction of these intermediate goals, not only as part of their preparation, but in the unhappy event that something goes awry with the marathon. I'm a positive person, but you have to consider the high-risk nature of this event; make sure you have a lot of positive experiences along the way.

Most of all, make sure the motivation to run a marathon is truly your own—not something you do only for family, friends, or social prestige. Don't decide to do it just because "everyone else does," or on a whim. The bottom line is that there's no better or more inspiring a goal than running a marathon, as long you're well-prepared and truly motivated for the right reasons.

These days, I find that a lot of first-timers either train with others or have been coached, and they are pretty realistic about their goals. I think that's because they are well informed. Some, like Wenche, do much better than they thought they would, because they didn't realize how different running the actual race is from training. Running along with others changes the nature of your effort, as does hearing the crowds cheer. But if what happened to Wenche happens to you and you run faster than you thought you would, let it be a surprise—because with modest goals you will stick to your vow to run sensibly. I promise you that if you take the advice in this book—if you are ready and run smart—you will feel what Wenche did, a great emotional high that began the minute she crossed the finish line and continues today.

One thing is for sure; you will never forget your first marathon. I never have. Because for me, without it, there would be no gold and silver World Championship and Olympic medals; there would be no travels around the world, or so many wonderful friendships.

THE MARATHON—AN EMOTIONAL EXPERIENCE

Many people run a marathon because they feel it is the ultimate in personal achievement, health, and fitness. They want to get in shape, or lose weight. They also do it for acceptance and status. From the minute you announce your intentions to run, you will receive a lot of approval, encouragement, respect, and even awe from others. Aside from getting in shape, probably the number one incentive for going the distance is emotional. People have overcome illness or other obstacles to run. In 1992, I coached New York City Marathon race director and friend Fred Lebow to his goal: running his own marathon while in remission from brain cancer, for his sixtieth birthday. I ran alongside him through the streets that year. As we entered Central Park, scores of people were waiting for him, cheering as loudly as they did for the winners. It was at that point I knew he was going to make it. With three miles to go, we embraced and burst into tears. It was the first time I ever cried in public. I was ecstatic for him because I knew how much this race meant to him. I never got my tenth victory in New York, but that day with Fred was another kind of victory. And it was such a different marathon experience from any of my others.

When you are fit, as I was, you take a lot of things for granted. That particular race opened my eyes to a different side of the event, one that I can most fully appreciate now as a cancer survivor myself. It makes me a lot more humble when I hear personal stories of those who have overcome hardships to complete the race. And sometimes, as you'll find, simply the achievement of going the distance is an emotional one. Every March, I stand at the finish line of the MORE Marathon for women in Central Park. The finishers cheer and embrace each other in tears. I have no idea why they are weeping, but then, neither did my co-author, Gloria. She was revisiting the distance after twelve years and ran it again at age 46. Even after working for the event for nearly two decades, it was as if it were new. To her utter surprise, she crossed the line and burst out crying.

Everyone has a reason to run. They are not all as dramatic as Fred's. They are often personal reasons, and likely emotional as well. But any reason that

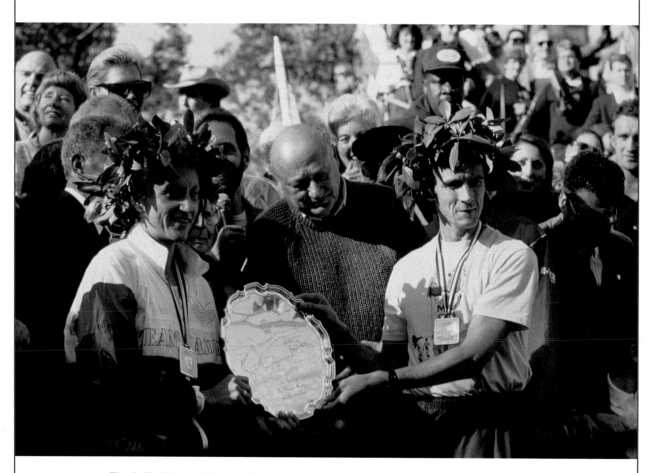

The thrill of victory. The awards ceremony after the 1988 New York City Marathon, one of my nine wins in that race.

gets you to the finish line is motivation enough. In most cases, you finish a marathon and you believe, "If I can do this, I can do anything."

I met Tim McLoone through the marathon circuit. He's a great guy. I don't know him so much as an athlete, but as a reporter and a musician. I read his son's blog about his battle with cancer every day, and my heart goes out to what he and his family are going through. As a runner himself, and one who has been in the pack for decades of television broadcasts, Tim knows better than most what the average marathoner goes through.

TIM McLOONE: I remember the famous Dr. George Sheehan describing his pre-running life: working, family, partying. Then he had what you could call a midlife crisis. He talked about beginning to run: It was like pulling the cord on the train that was taking him into oblivion. That was his metaphor. For a lot of people this is what it's like. Few drift into it. I don't think you're capable of running a marathon unless you make a conscious decision, because it's such an investment. Whether it's for weight loss or to control your own being, running becomes so elementary. Life revolves mostly around training for the race. I remember exactly when I realized marathoning had changed; it had become something for everyone. The starting gun went off at the Honolulu Marathon. About 1,000 people started running. The other 10,000 were walking.

As a lifelong competitive runner and, at the time, a television road race broadcaster for nearly a decade, I had heard all the platitudes: There are as many stories in the race as there are runners. In fact, I spent twenty years running those races, interviewing those people on live television. But one year, I had an epiphany, when I was struck by just how true the platitudes are. It was at the Los Angeles Marathon. I met a woman named Patsy Choco, whom the organizers said was a great cancer survivor story. She was strikingly nice, and that piqued my interest in her. It turned out she had entered the race two years earlier, but had to miss it to undergo a mastectomy. The next year, she missed it again, for a second mastectomy. The third year of the race, she found out the cancer had metastasized and she was terminal. She decided to discontinue her treatments, so she could train for and run that marathon.

Race day turned out to be a hot one. I was running through the crowds in a panic, trying to find Patsy among 20,000 other people. I finally spotted her two-thirds of the way through, surrounded by at least twenty-five people dressed in pink. She was suffering. We were coming to the end of the broadcast, and I finally got up the nerve to ask her, "Patsy, if you know that this is almost the guaranteed end of your life, why do it?"

"I know I'm going to die anyway," she answered. "But when my children look back, I want them to remember that their mom wasn't a quitter."

I stopped in my tracks. We were about to go off the air, and I signed off with the last line of the broadcast: "We are always obsessed with looking for heroes. Maybe we just aren't looking in the right place." There was a final camera shot of just her feet hitting the pavement. It was my moment of understanding that people run a marathon for their own reasons.

I look back at the marathons I've run, and I still can't believe I've done it. But I know exactly why I run. On November 10, 2006, when my young son, Jack, was diagnosed with leukemia, I drove out to the lake near where I live and went for a run that night. I guess I found some sort of release. There are a lot of extreme cases that inspire people to run, but most of us simply need to extract whatever force we can from ourselves. It all comes from within. That's the message for all of us.

2

Going the Distance

Once you contemplate running a marathon, let alone make the decision to run one, you need to understand exactly what it requires. Having the dream to run is one thing; having the health, the discipline, the time, and the know-how is yet another.

First of all, I'm sure what you've likely seen or heard is that anyone can get up off the couch and, with a couple of months of training, go the distance. It's not that simple. What I first said thirty-five years ago when I started running marathons still applies today: If you want to complete this race in any meaningful way, you are going to have to be reasonable about evaluating how much time and effort you are willing and able to devote.

In an ideal world, I believe a person starting from scratch, with no fitness base, should invest at least a year in preparing for a marathon. This is especially true if you are not an exerciser. But even if you are, the more time you allow yourself to prepare, the more miles you put in, the better the marathon you will run.

But ideals aside, on the minimum end of the time spectrum, a basically healthy person starting from scratch should allow at least six months (which is approximately the length of time it takes to complete the two programs in this book). What does it mean to start from scratch? The term "out of shape" needs to be clarified. There is "out of endurance shape," which means you aren't ready to run a long distance; "out of exercise shape," which means you're sedentary; and then there is a category for those with certain health conditions, such as being seriously overweight, or having a medical condition and/or risk of heart disease (e.g., high blood pressure). Not only should you consult a doctor before training if you have not done so already, but if you have health conditions, you should make a vow to take it especially slowly. The bottom line is that if you're a true beginner, you are going to have to walk before you can run. You can get to the marathon finish line; you just need to take your time doing it.

The beauty of running is it is universal. You don't need a special body type to run a marathon. Go out and watch any race, and you'll see as many body types as there are runners. They are short, tall, thin, or heavy. They bound along and they shuffle. So don't feel you need to go crazy with dieting to run a marathon. Being in shape doesn't mean you have to be slim. It's better to be a couple of pounds overweight and in good shape—as long as those pounds are cosmetic and not a health risk—than to be slim but unfit.

Another category to consider regarding going the distance is age, which is not as egalitarian as body size. I'm 52 now, but in my marathon prime I was 25. I know firsthand the difference in adapting to training as you age. Even though I am still in excellent physical fitness shape, progress is slower as I get older.

Generally, if you are over 40, your body needs more time to adjust to running higher mileage and the recovery is slower. However, as a person still physically active, I like to point out that age is somewhat relative. You can be any age and have a great fitness base, which puts you at a distinct advantage in your marathon preparation. Even though you might not have been a runner before deciding on a marathon, if you have a fitness background—from activities such as basketball, football, soccer, cycling, or working out in the gym—obviously you are at a better starting point than a person who has been sedentary. If you fit into this general fitness category, you can probably skip the beginner's program in the book.

The other advantage of being active before you undertake a marathon is that you may be better prepared not only physically, but also logistically and psychologically, because you are already programmed to exercise. Those new to exercising will not only have to make an activity change, but a lifestyle change as well. Trust me, though—once you do, there is no going back. Even after you cross the marathon finish line, I am confident that your race experience will ensure that you never want to go back to the "old days."

What outlook will you take when you decide to run? In my experience, a certain type (especially male) is more confident, even macho, in facing the unknown of the marathon. He's the kind of person who proclaims, "I can do this." I know this is a vast generalization, but when it comes to sports, men

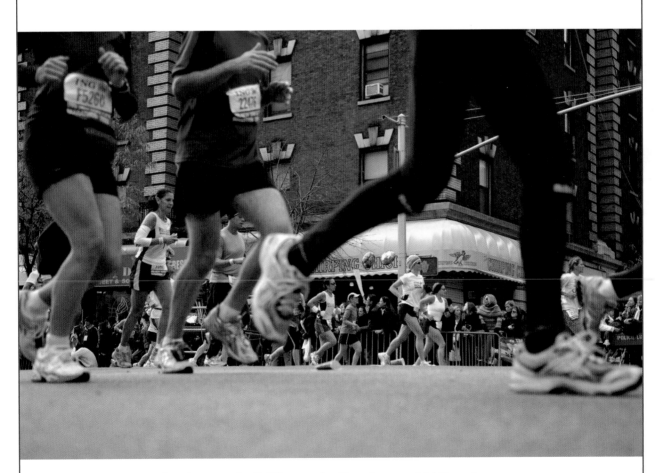

Running comes in all different styles. There is no one "right" way to run.

are usually more confident than women. (I hope with Title IX and changing attitudes, the next generation won't experience gender differences like this one.) I've met thousands of marathoners over the years. While I'm signing autographs at a marathon, a guy may come up to me and say, "I'm going to run 2:40." I always ask him for the details: *How* are you going to do that? I want to know. Is it just a boast, or can he back it up by telling me about his training and racing background? Most women who come up to me say, "I'm going to take my time. Nice and slow. I won't take any risks. I want to make sure I'm going to finish." They are also more inclined to look for reassurance, to express doubt and fear.

Trust me, you need great humility to run a marathon! While being a competitive person can be an advantage (I've found ambitious, competitive types have a greater chance of sticking to the program—challenging themselves to get better from one workout to the next), you don't want to be too intense or confident, or you may not be humble enough. If you are a person who lacks self-confidence, you will gain a greater sense of security as you move along in the program and experience success. You will overcome obstacles that you didn't think you could. You are taking control, reaching new heights, which will give you more confidence. Just make sure to build on this confidence by recognizing and acknowledging your interim achievements.

While physical health, and thus in some cases your readiness to run, might not be completely under your control, your attitude certainly is. In order to undertake the marathon journey, I firmly believe you have to be a positive person. That's because you will continually be challenged—not just to get through the miles, but in other aspects of the endeavor. You will be forced to find solutions: How will you find the time to train? What do you do when you don't feel particularly motivated? If you are a negative type, you may quickly find yourself defeated. You will say, "I can't get up at 6 a.m. to train." Or, "I'm not sure this is worth it." Whereas a positive person will say, "I want this goal. I will do what it takes. I will get up at 6 a.m. if necessary."

MAINTAINING YOUR BALANCE

Perhaps because they know I am very committed when I give my time, most of the people training for a marathon whom I have worked with have been very motivated. In fact, their intense enthusiasm and ambition often lead me to put things into perspective for them. I need to rein them in. I explain to them that they are not professional runners who simply eat, sleep, and train.

If you take on the marathon, you have to look at your training as a part of your whole life. Training for the marathon is one piece of a pie that includes other pieces, such as your job, your family, and your social obligations. Each part of the pie has an impact on the other. Planning your training depends on how your body feels, as well as what's going on at work or at home. It's often a delicate balance to fit everything together smoothly. Before I begin coaching someone, I make it clear that this balance must be in place for the program to

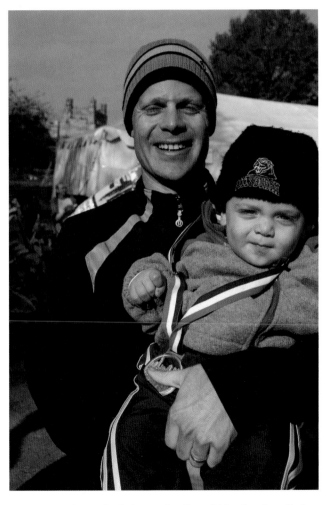

For the full marathon experience, include your family and friends—from finding an escort on a bicycle during your training runs, to meeting up after the big day to share a hug.

work. If training becomes overly stressful—you must constantly rush home to squeeze it in, for example—it transforms from a positive step toward a goal to being simply a burden. I am currently training a woman who recently missed one of her sessions due to a family event. She asked if she could make it up the following week, an equally busy time. "Forget about it," I told her, to let her off the hook.

Forcing the sessions into your life is when running becomes too great of an added stress. That's why I don't assign specific days for the workouts; that's for you to establish, according to what fits your schedule. Study the training program, understand it, and realize you may likely have to make some adjustments (such as not doing a hard run on a day you have other obligations or events).

The marathon goal shouldn't cause you to alienate coworkers, friends, or family. Don't run from people—literally. Training for the marathon shouldn't regulate, substitute for, or take over your life. Don't get me wrong. The marathon is a big deal, a great goal to work toward. It takes time and commitment. Just make sure that you both keep a healthy balance and know that the reason you are running is a positive one.

I think it helps keep perspective and balance when you share your experience. It inspires and motivates you to meet others with whom you share the marathon goal. Also, sharing your experience is a good way to pick up a lot of advice. (Just be careful, since you may suddenly encounter a lot of so-called "experts.") It is also helpful to study the marathon for yourself. Information and stories, as well as the specifics on the race you choose, are plentiful in books, magazines, and on the Internet. You will likely encounter a lot of conflicting information, but don't let that confuse you. There is no one way to train, no perfect plan to get from start to finish. That's why I've built a program with the foundation to get you ready and the flexibility for you to personalize it.

You need to be committed and well organized to train for a marathon. You will need to plan your daily and weekly workout schedule with care. You can't be all over the place. I've tried to coach "scattered" personalities before, and it hasn't worked out. I always stress that this kind of organization isn't drudgery; it's empowering. One of the great aspects of the marathon journey is the satisfying sense of order that structured training can give to your life. What I'm talking about is a basic commitment. But I have created a program that is flexible and reasonable. I understand that everyone occasionally gets ill, or that other unexpected events can interrupt training. While you don't have the luxury to take off three weeks, you may have to skip or rearrange a session or two.

From the minute you decide to run a marathon, it's going to be on your mind. Let it. That's part of the fun and excitement. But don't obsess over it. Before you spend significant time daydreaming about the "big day," start by focusing on short-term goals, like finishing a week of training, or completing one of the interim races.

Accept the ups and downs you will experience. You are going to have days you feel like you're flying and days you struggle. This is normal for all runners, not just first-timer marathoners. While I don't recommend pushing through serious pain, you may have days you have to overcome negativity. You might not feel like running, or you are upset or depressed. But it's worth it to persevere. In my and most other runners' experience, if you can coax yourself to go out and do the run, you'll feel better afterwards.

Finally, you don't have to have a special lifestyle to run a marathon. You don't have to rearrange your whole existence. You don't have to turn into a health nut and be in bed by 7:30 p.m. Of course, you shouldn't live on fast food and hit the pillow every night after midnight either. If you have to make too many lifestyle changes, though, the chances are you won't stick with the program. Just like the race, training is a long way to go. Have a smart journey!

There are so many stories of beginners (and even experienced runners) who underestimate the 26.2 miles. My husband, Jack, is one of them. Allan Steinfeld is another one. Allan was a master at helping to build marathons worldwide, but his bottom line message is a major theme of this book: respect the distance, and be prepared by doing your homework.

ALLAN STEINFELD: My road racing days date back to 1966, when the New York Road Runners (now the largest running organization in the world, which also conducts the New York City Marathon) used to hold just a few races for its 250 members. We would run on Sedgwick Avenue, right next to Yankee Stadium, and past all the broken-down cars and burned-out couches. I got to speaking with marathon pioneers, such as Joe Kleinerman and Ted Corbitt. At the time, the Boston Marathon had no hype, and no qualifying time. I was advised to send in a letter, and based on my other races, I was one of the 300 people accepted. We met at the schoolhouse at the start and had a physical exam. A doctor listened to our heart, basically to see if we were alive. He asked me, "Can you do it?" because I had never run a marathon before. I assumed I could run a pace a minute per mile slower than my eight-mile race time. That was fine for ten miles, but a few miles later I started breaking down, and at twenty-one miles, I couldn't move. I was getting cold, and there weren't many people around. I sat down on the ground and waved down a car. It pulled up, and the guy put the kids in the back, took a blanket from the trunk for me to wrap myself in, and drove me to the finish line.

What I learned from this experience is how difficult it is to run with no support along the course. Psychologically, it really makes a difference to have spectators cheer you on. When we were building the New York City Marathon, my boss at the New York Road Runners Club, Fred Lebow, said, "You can't bring the people to the marathon; you must bring the marathon to the people." And that's what's we did. After New York became so successful, we traveled around the country and the world, brought to major cities as advisors. We helped develop the same concept—bringing the race to the neighborhoods, making it a tour of the city. Today, you can run marathons like New York in London, Rome, Paris, Moscow, Beijing, Chicago, Los Angeles—just to name a few.

While the spectator crowds are great, all too often first-time marathoners get caught up in the hype. The adrenaline is pumping; they're flying high, and they just can't feel it, until it's too late. Stay on pace. Keep looking at your watch. You won't have any idea if you don't. And don't worry about how long it takes you. A lot of races have a long time limit. New York's is eight and a half hours, but the city only closes the streets to traffic for six and a half hours. Fortunately, there are sidewalks everywhere. When traffic opens up and the water stations have to close, we leave bottled water along the sidewalk for those people still running.

3
Getting Started

HURRY SLOWLY

My basic philosophy can be summed up by an expression we use in Norwegian: hurry slowly. Get there, but be patient. While I want you to reach your goal, and do it with focus and efficiency, I won't promise you the flashy "get fit quick" advice you will find advertised elsewhere. I want you to get there, but to do it smart; to do it right. There's making it to the finish line strong and triumphant, and then there's struggling to get there at all. And I want your marathon to be the start, not the finish, of your fitness. I also want you to be inspired to get the full experience—observe the miles adding up, do a race or two, make new friends. The goal is to get the most out of this lifetime experience.

My prescription to hurry slowly isn't just for psychological and emotional reasons. It is physical as well. Some people who start my training programs express surprise. They feel they are too slow. "Why aren't I breathing and sweating more, and more tired?" they ask. No matter which program you begin with, your body needs time to adjust—*all* of your body. Your joints, muscles, ligaments, etc., have to adapt to running, and that takes longer than your cardiovascular system. Think of yourself like a car. Your engine (your heart and lungs) may feel revved, but your wheels are rusty. You have to get the wheels lubricated, moving, and in gear. Trust me; by the time you do the long runs, you won't feel that the program is too slow. You will definitely know you are you getting a workout.

Hurry slowly is an expression you will see me use elsewhere in this book. It is a good one to remind yourself of during your training, as well as during your marathon.

WHAT IS FITNESS?

When I talk about fitness, I'm not just talking about the ability to run. Technically, fitness is a combination of endurance, strength, and flexibility. It is also a lifestyle, comprised of healthy habits. Although this is a book for an aspiring marathoner, it is my hope that while you get ready for going the distance, you also become physically fit—and inspired to maintain that fitness. In addition to being a great lifelong habit, the fitness I prescribe (using the strengthening and stretching exercises , as well as the nutritional advice in the book) will, in fact, also be your ticket to marathon success. Strength and flexibility are essential in creating the balance to running that will keep you injury-free, and good nutrition enables you to train properly and get through the race. So, I assure you, total fitness is an essential part of your training.

Fitness is also an attitude. It has become part of the way we live; how we eat, drink, and generally manage our lives. It includes exercise and healthy mental and psychological states of mind. Everybody talks about exercise and getting into shape. Obviously, by running a marathon, you will take that a big step further. Part of the benefit of the marathon experience is to recognize and gain the benefits of fitness, which you can maintain after the race is over. My motto is that it pays to get fit not because you get younger, but because you get older. It helps you to live better, for longer.

It's important to understand the exact nature of fitness, so you know where you stand for marathon preparation. Here is my breakdown of fitness levels:

Basic Fitness

If you walk up a set of stairs or go on a hike without getting winded, shovel snow for thirty minutes, play soccer or basketball with your children—if you are a sporadic exerciser, such as an occasional walker, who does a couple of exercise sessions a week, even if you miss a couple of sessions—you are what I term basically fit. You should start with my beginning running program before moving onto the marathon program to make sure you are "running fit." If, however, you find the rock bottom start of that program too easy, you can skip ahead until you find the right level—one which challenges you, but that still allows that vital time to get your muscles and joints used to road running. You'll know you've hit it right if your recovery from a session is reasonably short.

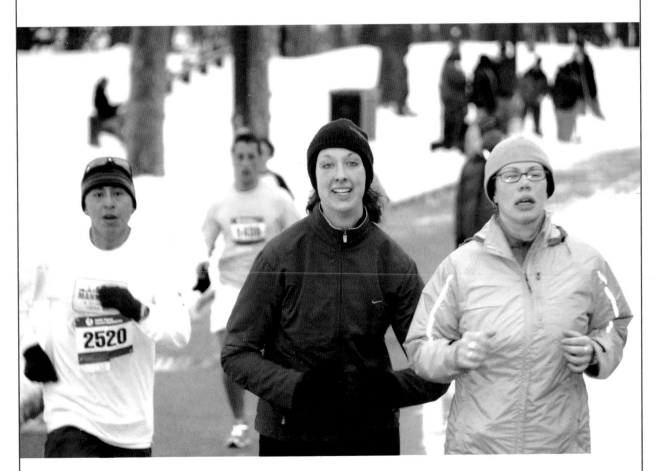

Running with friends, and in races, helps you get through the miles.

Optimal Fitness

If you have cardiovascular fitness, as well as some strength and flexibility—that is, if you do regular stretching exercises and some form of strength training, whether it is dedicated push-ups and sit-ups and/or weights, and you can run 5K (3.1 miles)—you are optimally fit; that is described as being "fit all over." And while this is an ideal state for health, it isn't enough to get you through 26.2 miles. You can skip the beginning running program, though, and start with the marathon program. That will get you to the next level, the third category of fitness.

Endurance Fitness

To make this relevant in terms of marathoning, I define this as follows: if you have the experience of training your body as a distance runner—you can run for one or two hours plus, your legs are used to "pounding the pavement," your muscles have been trained to optimally utilize glycogen (muscle fuel)—then you have endurance fitness. This is a specific fitness geared toward the marathon. You do not necessarily have optimal fitness, however. That is, you may be able to run a marathon and still not have the strength do ten push-ups or the flexibility to reach down and touch your toes.

If you are sedentary and want to lose weight, you are going to need patience. Although you may not have any health problems or risks, it may take you six months to get ready for a marathon. If you are already basically fit, it will take you less time: the four-month program is right for you. But you can't "cram" fitness. You can't do it all, every day. The stress/rest principle always applies (see Chapter 4).

Most of us who started running marathons "back in the day" got different advice than you get these days. Back in the early days of marathoning for the masses, aspiring participants used to be prescribed at least a year of running first, and often still are. I want to give you an idea of what I mean regarding patience, or rather, what it means when I say "hurry slowly." Of course, I am not prescribing my route to the marathon for you; I just want to illustrate the "layering" effect of training (and fitness) in my own career. Today, we have to create programs for endurance, strength, and flexibility. My background gave me those automatically.

I started running at about age 13 with Vidar, my sports club in Norway. We also did all sorts of other track and field activities (can you imagine me doing shot put? Well, I did! That develops overall fitness too). In a couple of years, I was running every day; three years later, I was running twice on most days, the program for serious distance runners. I maintained this mileage throughout my professional career: that's 80 to 100 miles a week from 1976 to 1990. I was fortunate to be injured only a couple of times in my entire career. Today, as a retired athlete (and proud "middle of pack" participant), I work out for forty-five minutes to an hour, most days of the week. I'm still a member of Vidar, where I began my lifelong exercise habit.

GETTING INTO THE HABIT

Since those early days, I've kept the fitness habit all my life. Even with the marathon goal to motivate you, you are still going to need to create a fitness habit. In the beginning, training may be tough. Being excited about running a marathon and deciding to do it is one thing. But there will come a point, I hope, when running, like anything else you do repeatedly, becomes a habit; when it seems as natural to you as going to work, or to shop and one day, ideally, as natural as brushing your teeth. When you experience what exercise does for you physically and mentally as you complete this marathon program, you are going to feel better about yourself. Maybe it will be your outlook; maybe you'll lose weight. You're going to go out to run, even if you're not in the mood, because you want that good feeling it gives you. And you'll know you're "hooked" when you come to a point when if you can't run for some reason, you miss it. You're physically and emotionally dependent on it.

You've already made the decision to "go the distance," but how can you reinforce the running habit? First off, find some support. It's easier to skip a run, breaking a date with yourself, than it is to break a date with a friend or a group. Most of the first-time marathoners I know train with others. In my career, eighty percent of my running was alongside training partners, either my husband Jack, or one of my two older brothers, Jan or Arild. Jack ran with me every morning for decades, and Jan or Arild did my afternoon hard training sessions with me. This was especially helpful, since it was often very hard for me to get out in the afternoons, when I was more tired. But I knew I had to meet my brothers.

It is helpful to create a routine for your training. Ask yourself some questions to fashion the best plan: Are you a morning or an evening exerciser? Do you like to run with friends or alone? Will you be able to train at the same time each day? When I was a teenager, I trained in the afternoons. But I didn't have the kind of responsibilities and distractions adults have—work, family,

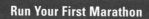

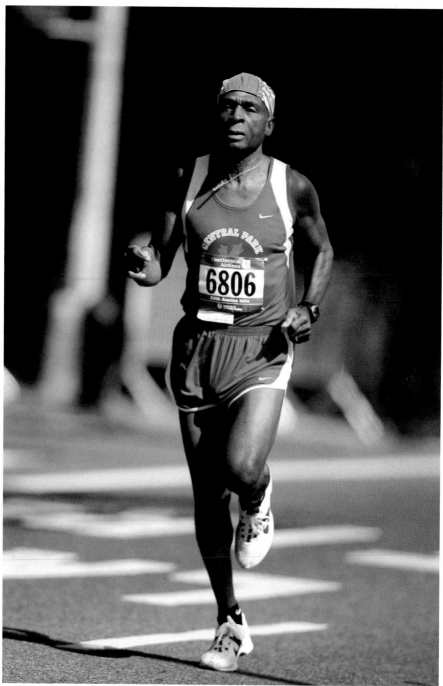

There will come a time when you can't believe you *weren't* a runner!

obligations, or potential emergencies. As I got older, I preferred to work out in the mornings. That is usually what I recommend, if you can do it. This way, you don't have to think about fitting it in later. And in my case, I'm lucky. Morning workouts are best for me. I'm not just a type A person; I'm an AAA. I'm very much awake extremely early in the morning and dead to the world by 5 p.m.

From a physiological perspective, the body is more warmed up and flexible in the afternoon (estimates are that at 4 p.m., bodies are in the ideal physical state for exercise). However, I feel people have a better chance of sticking to the program if they can train in the morning. While the downside is that you have to get up early, there are fewer potential distractions. You know your own lifestyle, but once the day gets going, you have to factor in everything that can pull you from your mission. It's also stressful if your training is weighing on your mind during the day. But the most important thing is to make the time, whether that means morning, afternoon, or evening.

So, set your alarm. If it helps motivate you, put your shoes and your clothes by the bed. Enlist your supporters. Have your running partner phone you or throw stones at your window if necessary. Make your spouse hold you to your running date. That will commit you. Don't be the kind of person who says, "I'll see how I feel tomorrow." You have to be very determined. Make a plan and stick to it. Over time, it becomes a habit.

THE WALK/RUN COMBINATION

Finally, you're almost ready to take off. But first, let's tackle the issue of running versus walking. Once upon a time, the only way to do a marathon was to run one, or at least jog. Walking meant defeat, as it was often the last resort of a runner who had slowed down. Many experts these days feel that, to the contrary, walking is not only allowable, but that walking breaks are well advised. And they prescribe walking even for experienced marathoners. They claim that's because greater running effort can cause you to feel heavy-legged. A combination of walk/run helps to avoid, or lessen, the chemical reaction that causes muscles to get stiff. I've come around to this way of thinking myself, particularly for beginners. I saw how well it worked for my sister-in-law in her first marathon. Two years ago, I met John Stanton, founder of the Running Room in Canada, at the Ottawa Marathon. In my opinion, his training ideas about running and walking make a lot of sense. First of all, I like the fact that he stresses two aspects in his beginning marathon advice: the program should be gentle and progressive. By gentle, he means that the program should be comfortable and safe, designed to help you stay motivated and injury-free. Progressive means that it gets you to improve. The third part of his plan goes without saying: have fun.

Stated basically, the goal of endurance training, or, in this case, long, slow distance running, is to keep you on your feet, adapted to being out on the roads. Stanton feels that the run/walk combination extends the distance you can run. Run/walk follows the similar principle of hard/easy. It also distributes the workload to various muscles, thus potentially helping to delay fatigue. Stanton feels that walking also facilitates "stretch breaks." A brisk walk creates a stretch that extends throughout the entire lower body. Physical and mental variety is always a good prescription in training, and the run/walk combination provides that variety.

In both training and the race, the most important thing is to cover the distance. If you feel you the need to walk periodically, do so. If you use this technique in either training or racing, my only advice is to take the walking breaks early, before you feel you really need them. When you begin to walk only after you feel like you can't run anymore, you will run an overall slower time than those who distribute their energy by taking walking breaks earlier. For example, taking a three-minute walk every mile results in a faster time than walking the last six miles of the race because you're "done in." That's simple math. As Stanton points out, the average runner will lose less than 10 seconds per kilometer by doing run/walk rather than all running. The person running continuously, but fatiguing, will slow down much more than 10 seconds a kilometer by the end of the run.

Obviously, if you can run the entire marathon (or training run), that's fine. Some people feel disoriented by shifting from run to walk; some feel if they walk, they won't get running again. And some simply feel the training prepares them sufficiently to run the entire distance.

COACHING

I had coaching throughout my career, but eventually I knew what to do for myself. Some people want a coach, and it can be a great benefit. If you feel you need someone to more closely advise you, as well as to keep you on track, it's fine to hire a personal trainer or a coach. Just be aware that it will cost you, and that prices can be steep. There is a range of services you can purchase, from advice to a coach who is also a running partner. Less expensive options are Internet coaching, in which an expert counsels you via email. Ask around for recommendations by contacting your local running club or organization. Not every coaching situation is a formal one, however. You can get informal coaching advice from experienced runners, such as those who work in running specialty stores or who compete for running clubs.

CHOOSING A MARATHON

Perhaps you already have a marathon in mind, or a specific race is your incentive to run. Some people are so inspired by watching an event that they sign up to do it themselves. Or they have friends or family members who have done a specific marathon, and they want to do the same one. And some simply choose a race for convenience, because it is nearby. There are many questions you should ask yourself before choosing which marathon to run and a variety of factors to take into consideration. Since this event will be a landmark for you, it is important to make the best possible choice, which means it should be well thought out.

One question is whether you'd like to make a trip out of the experience and so pick a distant destination. Is cost a factor? Will you fly, or is a long drive the extent of your willingness to travel? Or are you more comfortable staying close to home, where the commitment is less drastic and which may be easier? Certainly, negotiating travel, possible weather or even time zone changes, and eating and sleeping in an unfamiliar spot is a risk. On the other hand, a marathon can be a good rationale for a trip and also an exciting part of the marathon adventure. While you'll want to save your legs and delay sightseeing until after your race, having a new place to visit can also give you reason to run. In the final analysis, if you are careful and educated about your choice of destinations, your risks from running out-of-town are no greater than you would incur in any marathon.

Consider the many that have gone before you. Almost every one of the thousands of first-time marathoners I meet is looking for a lifetime experience. They're not just in it to cover the distance. That's why I advise you to choose a place and a race that will really get you psyched up. Perhaps I'm prejudiced, since all of my marathon experiences were in major races, but my feeling is backed up by the thousands of other marathoners I've met. Personally, I feel that one of the incentives of training is to get you to a big event, one with all the fanfare, which often occur in a major city or at a major race, such as one of the theme races, like the Rock 'n' Roll marathons. I've been to marathons of every size and shape, all over the world, and I feel strongly that you will greatly benefit by the excitement of having other runners around you and a crowd of spectators to cheer you on (and maybe even music along the course, like in many big races), as opposed to a race in which you can run for an hour without seeing another person. It is easy for people to be super-motivated and excited when they are drawn into the talk of races like New York, Chicago, or Los Angeles. In fact, everyone I speak with usually wants London or New York to be his or her first marathon experience. Especially if they are going to do it only once, they want to run one of "the classics." You don't have to go overseas, though, if that is too much of an investment. There are plenty of races that meet this description in every corner of the United States.

As unfounded as it usually turns out to be, a common first timer's fear is coming in last. They don't want to feel "exposed," the way you can in a smaller race. However, in a big crowd, you can disappear. You won't feel like you are on display. Although obviously I was always exposed in the races I ran, I recognize the benefits of being part of the pack. In addition to New York, I ran Stockholm, London, and Boston. The only times I ran with fewer than thousands of others were at the World Championships and the Olympics, but there were still a lot of people cheering us on along the course and obviously, because of the stature of those events, an atmosphere of excitement.

However, if the idea of all the hoopla ties you up in knots, or it's just not your thing, by all means, choose a smaller race. Also, there are plenty of possible themes from which to choose. If combining a marathon with a love of history or tradition is appealing, there are races like Charlottesville, in Virginia, or the Marine Corps Marathon in Washington, D.C. Hawaii might motivate you—or the redwoods of the Big Sur International Marathon in California.

An important factor for almost any race you choose is timing. It has to fit into both the most optimal part of your schedule and the most optimal running season. Usually marathons are scheduled during moderate seasons to avoid extreme weather, and while they are run on a variety of terrains—from the wide, flat streets of Chicago or Los Angeles to the hilly countryside of Vermont—make sure you know the type of terrain you are choosing and that you will be able to train in similar circumstances. Some marathons I have run are on flat terrain, but not all (such as New York, with rising areas over bridges and some winding turns, or the famously hilly Boston).

Timing applies especially to signing up for a race. If you do choose a major marathon like New York or Chicago, you will need to enter well ahead of time, usually at least six months. And various races—from New York to Big

Sur—are very hard to get into, so in addition to exploring them early, you will want to have an alternative race lined up if you don't get in.

Here is some further advice on selecting a marathon, based on the priorities of my dear friend, the late New York City Marathon race director Fred Lebow.

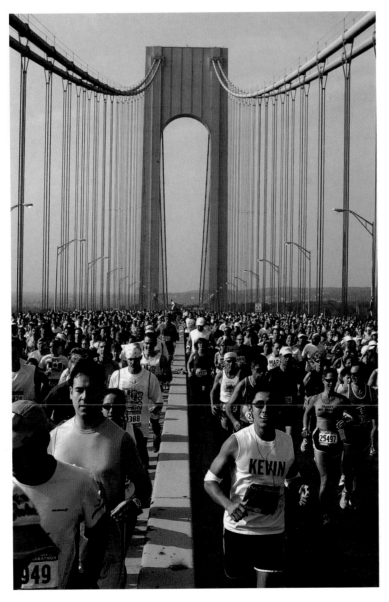

The famous New York City Marathon in the first mile on the Verrazano-Narrows Bridge.

Fred not only built the New York race, but also helped to develop major marathons around the world. He also ran a remarkable sixty-nine marathons himself, so he really knew what he was talking about.

Talk to the veterans: Ask friends or acquaintances about the races they have chosen, what they recommend, and why. The greater the number of people you can speak with and the more experience they have, the better. Revisit them for further tips once you select a race.

Travel wisely: You should choose a race to which you can travel fairly easily, i.e., fly to directly or drive. Make sure your lodging is near the start and/or finish, or that there is special transportation (such as buses) for the runners. Hassling with getting to the start drains your physical and mental energy, which can be better used for the run, and searching for friends and relatives and/or a ride back after the race is especially difficult when you are cold and tired.

Make sure your race is well-organized: The course should advertise itself as "certified," and it should have frequent mile or kilometer markers and clocks or split timers (people calling out times). There should be numerous water and aid stations. (Major marathons have them at every mile). There should be some medical personnel. Find out if sports drinks or gels will be available, so you will know to practice ingesting them in your training and/or be prepared to bring your own.

Expo: It's a nice plus if the race has an Expo (Exposition), a running specialty fair with exhibitors, product sampling, demonstrations, and guest speakers. This is part of the ambience of the event, like a pre-race pasta party, which is another nice addition.

I always looked at the profile of my marathons (on their Web site and/or on the race application, or I made sure to be advised) to see what kind of courses they were run on and what services they offered. It was important to know if I faced some special challenges. That dictated the way I might structure my training. However, I wasn't always as briefed as I should have been, and this turned out to make all the difference in at least one crucial case. I was told all about the infamous Heartbreak Hill in Boston. In fact, there are three or four hills before you even get to the big one. I even trained on them before the race. What I didn't factor in was this: what goes up must come down. What killed me in that race was all the downhill running, including the entire first mile. By the time I got to Heartbreak Hill, I was actually relieved to being going *up*, to rest my legs from all the downhill pounding. Now, I always tell people, especially those focused on the effort of going uphill, not to underestimate the impact on the legs of downhill running. Also, when people ask me about a course, I give them an overview of the *entire* race. For example, I advise people running New York to save energy for the second half of the race, which has more inclines than the first half, yet most people don't realize that. The bottom line message from my Boston experience is obvious: Make sure you know as much as possible about the entire route, not just the general layout or a few notable parts.

People often ask if they should try to train on some of the actual race courses. It's nice, but not necessary. In my case, in the spring I ran part of the course in Los Angeles before the 1984 Summer Olympics. It was helpful in the psychological sense, because it gave me something to visualize in my training. But I didn't run the course at all before the World Championships in Helsinki, and I had a great race there. It's not often possible to test the actual race course, especially if you're traveling to the event. What's more important is to study everything you can about the event.

WALK-TO-RUN BEGINNING PROGRAM

This is an excellent program to begin your marathon training, if you are starting from scratch. From it, you can safely, sensibly, and confidently build your base for the big event. You may be under the impression that all running programs are meant to make you breathe hard and sweat. That's a myth. Initially, the goal is to familiarize yourself with the activity and make it a comfortable one. To get you to the marathon, your body, mind and lifestyle must undergo the necessary adaptation, and education. This program is a perfect introduction.

I have been prescribing this program (which I customized for this book, to make it optimal for marathon preparation) since 1990 to thousands of people ranging in ages from their twenties to their sixties, including students, senior citizens, and corporate groups. In fact, many of the 45,000 women who for many years participated annually in the Grete Waitz Run, which I conducted in Norway, utilized this program. The way I see it, if it worked for all of these people, it will work for you!

PROGRAM

Week 1

Day 1	Day 2	Day 3
Walk 5 min.	Walk 5 min.	Same as Day 2
Jog 1 min./walk 1 min. × 6	Jog 1 min./walk 1 min. × 7	Same as Day 2
Walk 5 min.	Walk 5 min.	Same as Day 2
22 min. total	24 min. total	24 min. total

Week 2

Day 1	Day 2	Day 3
Walk 5 min.	Same as Day 1	Same as Day 1
Jog 1 min./Walk 1 min. × 4		
Jog 2 min./Walk 2 min. × 2		
Jog 1 min./Walk 1 min. × 2		
25 min. total		

Week 3

Day 1	Day 2	Day 3
Walk 5 min.	Same as Day 1	Same as Day 1
Jog 3 min./Walk 2 min. × 4		
Jog 4 min.		
Walk 2 min.		
31 min. total		

Week 4

Day 1	Day 2	Day 3
Walk 5 min.	Walk 5 min.	Same as Day 2
Jog 5 min.	Jog 6 min.	Same as Day 2
Walk 3 min.	Walk 3 min.	Same as Day 2

Jog 7 min.	Jog 6 min.	Same as Day 2
Walk 5 min.	Walk 3 min.	Same as Day 2
Jog 5 min.	Jog 4 min.	Same as Day 2
Walk 4 min.	Walk 3 min.	Same as Day 2
34 min. total	30 min. total	30 min. total

Week 5

Day 1	Day 2	Day 3
Walk 5 min.	Walk 5 min.	Same as Day 1
Jog 4 min./walk 1 min. × 2	Jog 7 min.	Same as Day 1
Jog 8 min.	Walk 2 min.	Same as Day 1
Walk 2 min.	Jog 5 min./walk 1 min. × 2	Same as Day 1
Jog 6 min.	Jog 8 min.	Same as Day 1
Walk 2 min.	Walk 2 min.	Same as Day 1
33 min. total	36 min. total	33 min. total

Week 6

Day 1	Day 2	Day 3
Walk 5 min.	Walk 5 min.	Same as Day 1
Jog 7 min./walk 2 min. × 2	Jog 10 min.	Same as Day 1
Jog 8 min.	Walk 3 min.	Same as Day 1
Walk 2 min.	Jog 8 min.	Same as Day 1
Jog 3 min.	Walk 2 min.	Same as Day 1
Walk 2 min.	Jog 6 min.	Same as Day 1
	Walk 2 min.	
38 min. total	36 min. total	38 min. total

Week 7

Day 1	Day 2	Day 3
Walk 5 min.	Same as Day 1	Same as Day 1
Jog 12 min.	Same as Day 1	Same as Day 1
Walk 2 min.	Same as Day 1	Same as Day 1
Jog 8 min./walk 1 min. × 2	Same as Day 1	Same as Day 1
37 min. total	37 min. total	37 min. total

Week 8

Day 1	Day 2	Day 3
Walk 5 min.	Same as Day 1	Same as Day 1
Jog 15 min.	Same as Day 1	Same as Day 1
Walk 2 min.	Same as Day 1	Same as Day 1
Jog 15 min.	Same as Day 1	Same as Day 1
Walk 3 min.	Same as Day 1	Same as Day 1
40 min. total	40 min. total	40 min. total

Week 9

Day 1	Day 2	Day 3
Walk 5 min.	Same as Day 1	Same as Day 1
Jog 20 min.	Same as Day 1	Same as Day 1
Walk 2 min.	Same as Day 1	Same as Day 1
Jog 10 min.	Same as Day 1	Same as Day 1
Walk 3 min.	Same as Day 1	Same as Day 1
40 min. total	40 min. total	40 min. total

Week 10

Day 1	Day 2	Day 3
Walk 5 min.	Same as Day 1	Same as Day 1
Jog 30 min.	Same as Day 1	Same as Day 1
Walk 5 min.		
40 min. total	40 min. total	40 min. total

For the runs during the last two weeks, you need not walk first. Start the jog slowly instead to warm up.

Week 11

Day 1	Day 2	Day 3
Jog 40 mins.	Same as Day 1	Jog 45 mins.

Week 12

Day 1	Day 2	Day 3
Jog 45 mins.	Jog 50 mins.	Same as Day 2

4
The Training

UNDERSTANDING WHAT TO EXPECT

I think the basic question for any prospective marathoner is how to prepare to enter "no man's land." As efficient as training can be, it cannot wholly prepare you. This is uniquely true to marathoning because you do not run the entire distance in training, but it is also true of all training, which can never exactly duplicate a race. First of all, how will you know what to expect? What should the training feel like? For each and every first-timer, the marathon is a mystery until you've had the experience. My goal is to demystify it as much as possible, to teach you to speak the "marathoner's language."

While training can't duplicate the true marathon experience, if you pay close attention, it can educate you on the many ups and downs you will likely face. This is particularly true during your long runs, when you should note

41

what phases you go through, both physically and mentally. I guarantee you, no matter who you are, you're going to have good and bad days, like every experience in life. This is a universal truth in marathoning, whether you're a beginner or a world-class runner. In all my years of running marathons, this roller coaster ride never ended. So, it helps to understand and accept it as part of the process. However, experience teaches us how to negotiate this ride. For example, sometimes you'll hit a low, and you may assume it's because you're not in shape, or you're troubled or distracted by something else in your life, which is interfering with your training. But it can also be something as simple as low blood sugar that gives you the "running blahs." In other words, in some instances you can fix the problem quickly, or it may be something that takes time and experience to solve. This is why keeping a diary and consulting experienced runners is particularly helpful.

What about the positive side of the equation, when you finish a training run and feel it was perfect? You'll want to duplicate that experience as much as possible, of course. Part of the basic appeal of running goes back to the decades-old cliché of getting a "runner's high." It's often defined as the feeling of effortlessness, in which time and space seem to dissolve and everything happens magically. It's as close to being in the moment as possible. In short, you feel great.

I've never personally experienced the so-called "runner's high." Maybe that's because even though it's out of fashion, the term suggests a drug high, and I've never taken drugs. But the expression has come to define a certain state of mind. While you will meet marathoners who struggled, at least for a time, you will undoubtedly all meet marathoners who experienced the perfect race and felt the emotions of a "runner's high."

While I wouldn't call it a "high," I have had what I would call the perfect race. And it was an unforgettable experience. It happened most notably in the inaugural World Championships Marathon in Helsinki in 1993. I felt that I was in complete control and that whatever happened, I could respond. If the pace picked up, I could handle it; if the leaders took off, I could go with them. I felt confident. I never struggled with the effort, or felt any pain. When I crossed the finish line victorious, arms raised in the air in happiness, I could have kept on running if I had to.

There are days you feel invincible. Keeping track of the details of your training in a running diary will hopefully help you to duplicate the experience (right).

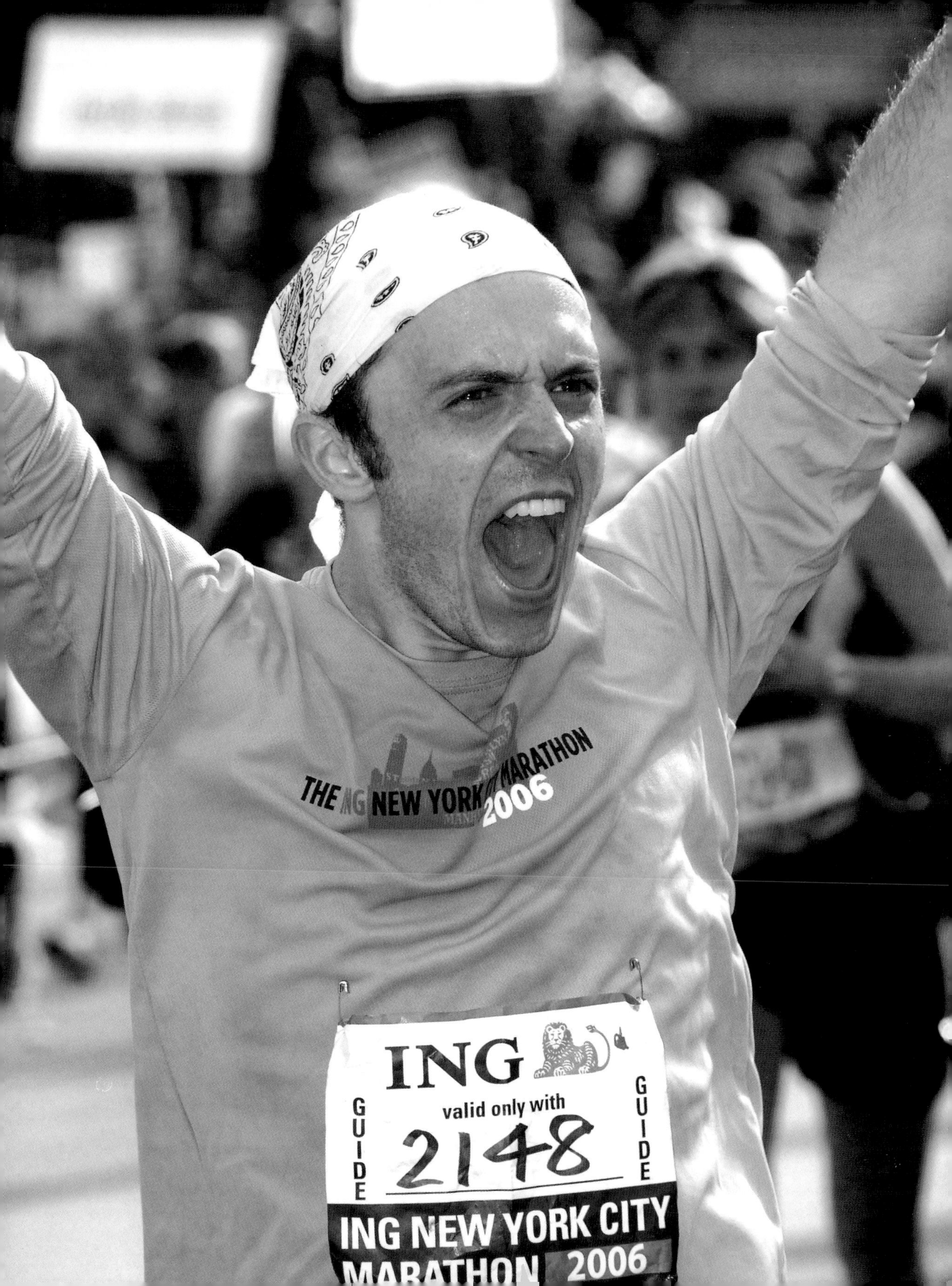
THE ING NEW YORK CITY MARATHON 2006
ING
GUIDE
valid only with
2148
GUIDE
ING NEW YORK CITY
MARATHON 2006

I'm sure you would love to have this experience, and it's possible. However, understand that an athlete has a perfect race maybe once or twice in a career. And when you have the experience, you try to bottle that formula, to copy it. I tried to do that in my next race, to recreate what had produced such magic in the previous marathon. Despite my best efforts, however, the next race was hard work all the way. I won the New York City Marathon nine times, and frankly, not one of them came easily. That doesn't mean they weren't satisfying. My point is that it's okay to listen to other people's inspiring stories and to admire them. And it's okay to seek the perfect race. But when you sign up to run a marathon, you accept that it takes work to prepare for it and effort to get through it. After all, if a marathon were easy, everyone would do it. And then, what would be the challenge?

While you may not be able to guarantee the ideal experience, I do believe you can train yourself to successfully face down and conquer the challenges you may encounter. My experiences are similar to most every marathoner I've met or trained. You've simply got to accept the cycles. I've been five miles into a marathon and felt my legs getting heavy. "How will I ever make it to the end?" I asked myself. But at ten miles, I felt great again. Of course, you don't know what will ultimately happen; I didn't know those bad patches would pass, but I had faith they would, based on my training. Training prepares you to be as ready as possible for anything in the race.

You may have days when you doubt yourself and days when you feel you could go on for many more miles (but don't!). You can expect certain physical cycles as well. You may experience some aches and pains during or after training. A feeling of fatigue or general soreness can be natural, but if it lasts longer a week, perhaps the program is moving too quickly for you, or the pace you are running is too fast. For the most part, if you have a base of fitness when you begin, and if you follow the program, you should feel pretty good most of the time. But don't be afraid to make adjustments if physical discomfort persists.

You may go through an array of experiences in training, and, forewarned, you will recognize them if they crop up again. You will learn how to stay calm and work through them. But as I've said, even the best training cannot completely prepare you for the actual race. All my training indicated that I was in the best shape of my life approaching my one try at the Boston Marathon, yet it ended up being the worst marathon of my career. On the other hand, I've run my marathon race pace in training for a mere eight miles and been exhausted. "How can I keep this up for 26.2 miles?" I wondered. But that was before I tapered and rested in the final pre-race week, before I felt the adrenaline and nervous anticipation of the start, saw the people, and heard the sounds of the helicopters and loud speakers. Then, I was like a horse in the starting gate. Truly born to run!

This magic feeling is attainable, and it can happen in your first marathon. Even though you will be ready for anything and everything, in the best-case scenario you might be one of the fortunate ones who simply flies and has the race of a lifetime.

Here are some important training principles to keep in mind:

HARD/EASY

All training programs, for all levels of runners, follow the principle of hard/easy. This is the system in which a strenuous effort is followed by rest—in this case, indicated in the training programs by a day (or days) off. It is not just the miles you run, but how they are distributed that will make your training most effective. Running is hard on your legs. Without the rest, you risk injury, and you can't absorb the benefits of training. Also, the mental break is important, particularly for the novice. With rest, the body rejuvenates itself, on both a physical and mental level.

RUNNING SURFACES

A decade of track running ensured that I trained a relatively modest amount on hard surfaces (i.e., asphalt or concrete) for the first part of my career. Although I did not completely avoid the roads, I had the balance of running on softer surfaces. Marathoning changes that equation, since it is likely that all, or most, of your training will be done on hard surfaces. It is actually necessary, in order for your legs to adapt to the pounding you will experience in the race. However, you can balance the stress of running on hard surfaces by doing some of your training on softer surfaces. Just be careful with your footing, as some softer surfaces tend to be uneven (such as grass or trails) and can potentially cause another set of problems. Also, try to avoid heavily crowned (sloped) roads, or make sure to run equal distances on opposite sides of a crowned road.

Running Surfaces (Rated by *Runner's World* from Best to Worst)

1. Grass
2. Wood Chips
3. Dirt
4. Cinders/Decomposed granite
5. Synthetic Track

6. Treadmill
7. Asphalt
8. Sand
9. Concrete (approximately ten times harder than asphalt)
10. Snow

THE MARATHON FOR THOSE OVER 40

If you're running a marathon and you're over 40, you're far from alone. In fact, according to the most recent statistics from Running USA's Road

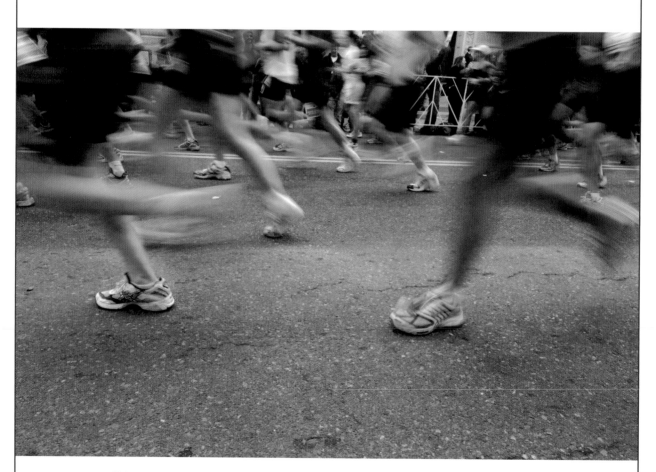

Take care to train smart. Up to 70 percent of running injuries are of the lower leg (and feet), and related to the biomechanics of the feet.

Running Information Center, 46 percent of U.S. marathoners in 2006 were masters—that is, over age 40. With the exception of getting a medical checkup if you have not done so, there is no built-in age difference for the training I prescribe. However, if you have little or no athletic background, you should probably allow a cushion of extra time between the start of your training and the race date (say, seventeen or eighteen weeks) so that you may comfortably repeat a week or two if necessary, since aging can delay recovery.

Although an older runner usually takes longer to recover from efforts and from injury, it is worth considering another aspect of age. In running circles, we talk

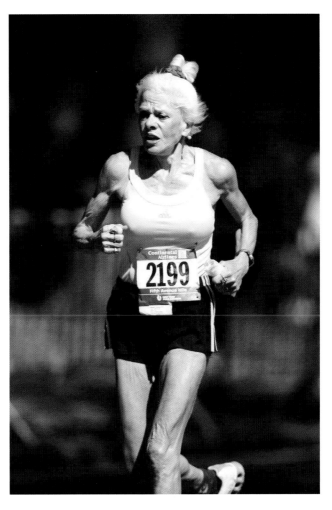

Running is remarkably versatile. You can find the "athlete within" at any age.

about two kinds of ages, the chronological age and the "running age." If you've met experienced runners over age 40 that complain they are more frequently injured, it doesn't necessarily mean it is strictly an age-related problem. It could likely be the result of the accumulation of miles over the years. By this measure, a twenty-five-year-old who has been running since high school is much "older" than a novice forty-year-old. Take note, young runners! On the plus side, an older runner may be better able to use general experience and life wisdom to take a more "common sense," and thus more successful, approach to the marathon.

TREADMILLS

In general, it is best to do the bulk of your training outdoors, because it more closely duplicates what you will experience in the race. Also, part of the experience of running is being outside and enjoying or negotiating the elements and your surroundings. That being said, if weather, time of day (specifically, the risks of running in the dark), or convenience necessitates using a treadmill, by all means do so. Although I did most of my workouts on the roads, I did do some running on a treadmill. An example was my very early morning runs, because of traffic and darkness. Be aware, however, that when you run on a treadmill, it employs a different action (and thus different muscles) than running on the roads. You are not pushing off on a treadmill, because it is moving. You just lift your legs. You don't use energy to go forward, like you do outdoors. On the other hand, you get the same cardiovascular benefits on a treadmill and fewer of the potential negative effects of pounding, since you run on a softer, more forgiving surface. So if you're coming off a long run, for example, a treadmill can be a relief for tired or sore legs. You can also control such variables as speed and incline.

There are a couple of other things to know about the treadmill. If you aren't familiar with one, take the time to learn how it works and to test it, and adapt to it with shorter runs or walks. When you get comfortable with the machine, vary the speed and incline to distribute the stress on the body and/or to duplicate outdoor terrain (a one to two percent incline is generally recommended, which better duplicates the roads). Since there is no wind resistance when you run on a treadmill, you'll heat up very quickly, so make sure to run with a fan or some ventilation. You'll perspire more, so stay well hydrated. If you are contemplating purchasing a treadmill, be aware that the most expensive models are not always the ideal. Do some homework, including testing out the machines before you buy, if possible.

HAND OR LEG WEIGHTS

Often you see runners or walkers with hand or even ankle weights. They believe they get a better workout by increasing their workload. However, physical therapist and sports injury expert Gerard Hartmann does not believe there is a physiological benefit from carrying weights when you run. First of all, it changes your natural cadence; secondly, it can be dangerous, because it changes your natural gait, which can lead to injury. Doing the strengthening exercises in Chapter 7 is a better bet to achieve your goals than carrying weights while you work out.

HEADSET AND IPOD

While you may choose to use either of these devices on a treadmill, I am not a fan of using them outdoors, largely because of the safety risk. You cannot be fully aware of your surroundings—terrain, traffic, or other people—when you are plugged into a headset. Most running clubs and organizations also advise against their use outdoors. If you do insist on using them outdoors, keep the volume turned very low (lower than your usual) and take one out one of the earpieces. Also, I feel you should not consider wearing them in a race. (In fact, some races prohibit it for safety reasons.) You want to totally immerse yourself in the race experience—and everything happening around you. In shorter races, you will be practicing for your marathon, and you need your focus. In the actual marathon, you'll want to soak up the atmosphere and focus on everything you need to run well. If you feel the urge for distraction, such as during training, find a partner so you can chat during your run. You can always listen to music after the training run or race, relaxing on the couch.

5

The Marathon Training Program

ABOUT THE PROGRAM

Some people misunderstand or underestimate the marathon. They see their friends or associates do it, "average" people who don't look like runners. They automatically think, "If he can do it, I can do it." Unless they are superhuman, I guarantee you that all "average" runners followed a serious training program.

Not that long ago, the marathon was an event undertaken by only a handful of serious competitive athletes. It's a terrific trend that today thousands of others, including those who would consider themselves non-athletes, have succeeded in going the distance. But one trend I don't agree with is the many claims for get-fit-quick programs, promising to prepare you for a marathon in record time. Even the most minimal program should be constructed to give you a solid foundation and the confidence to know you will be well prepared if you follow it.

As with every general fitness program, there is no such thing as "one size fits all." You may need to adjust (personalize) this one as you progress. The program is intended for sixteen weeks, but as I advise throughout the book, try to build in a several-week cushion of extra time before your marathon. After all, let's face it, life intervenes. Four months is a long time to go without a single potentially disruptive incident—a cold, the flu, family obligations, or work emergency—that could interrupt your training. Those who are over 40, or just feel the need, may find they are better off taking more time (e.g., they might repeat week eight) to complete the program. And remember, you can still get injured if you are 25.

You may "fall off the wagon," or have to cross train and miss some running. While it may not affect the overall result to miss one or two of the shorter sessions, missing a long run would make it unlikely you are totally prepared for the marathon. And if you are lucky enough that everything does go right and you finish the program in sixteen weeks, you can easily repeat week fifteen and be fine. For others, the opposite may be true. You may feel the program is slow and that you could "push the envelope." My advice is not to. Rather, celebrate the feeling (and, I hope, the reality) that you have everything under control. Remember the Norwegian motto I use: Hurry slowly.

In that vein, you have to "walk before you can run." You should be able to run at least three miles before beginning this program. If you aren't yet at that level, start with the beginning program in Chapter 3.

THE LONG RUNS

The program is designed to build up your longest runs slowly, thus safely. When running long, most experts seem to agree with John Stanton, who claims that the number one mistake beginners make is to push the pace for the first three to four miles and then try to continue with that intensity. All the runs should be done at an aerobic, or comfortable, pace (using heart rate as a guide. See Chapter 6). LSD (long slow distance) should be just that, as you adapt your body to being on the roads for a given length of time. Stanton points out that if you start slow and keep the pace steady, by the fourth or fifth week you'll feel stronger and automatically start running faster. As I say elsewhere in the book, while you can keep track of how long you're out, don't make time the focus of your running.

Long runs accomplish several things. When you are out on the roads two hours or more, your body depletes its glycogen stores (energy, in the form of carbohydrates). At that point, the body begins to draw on its fat stores. Training makes your body adapt to this necessary shift and gets it ready for the race. Also, when you deplete the glycogen stores several times, the body compensates by learning how to store more glycogen in the muscles. In essence, you become a better "sponge." Thus, practicing the long runs makes you a more efficient runner overall.

You will experience certain changes during the long runs and learn to recognize what you can expect in the actual race. You may feel some lows and then come out of them, and, while you want to do the "form check" recommended by John Stanton (see below), as your body fatigues, your stride may naturally shorten as you run slower. Don't get caught up in that, or in any one cycle or feeling. The same holds true for any one training session. Keeping track of your experiences in a diary will help you to recognize the various cycles and understand that not every training run is exactly the same.

You may encounter some programs or advocates who recommend running the entire 26.2 miles in training, to make sure you can do it. However, my philosophy is the more common one found in most training programs: If you can run eighteen to twenty miles in training, when it comes to the actual race, the tapering you've done, coupled with the atmosphere of the race, will carry you through the extra six miles. Also, there is a downside to going the entire distance in training. You will need a long time to recover from it; you may be discouraged, since it will likely be slower and more difficult than the actual race; and you could injure yourself. Also, I think psychologically there is some risk of burning out, or peaking too soon.

Some people measure their run by time—making sure they are on their feet for three or more hours. You can run for a given time if you prefer, or if it's difficult to mark off the miles. It isn't mandatory to run by miles, but if you do, it isn't important whether it's exactly 18 or it turns out to be 17 ½ miles. For the purpose of a general training program, it is easier to prescribe the runs in miles, as most people are miles-oriented.

TRAINING FACTORS

As for running surfaces, keep in mind that you are training to most accurately duplicate the actual marathon. My sister-in-law Wenche did a portion of her training on the soft surface of the trails near her home. That was good to save her legs from pounding, but I advised her to eventually do some of the long runs on the roads, to prepare her legs to undergo what they would have to in the race. (See Running Surfaces in Chapter 4.)

As with the beginning program in the book, this one focuses on training only a few days a week. Even if you feel you can run more often, as the runs get longer and harder, you'll realize that you will need the days off to recover, to be fresher for the next session. You should adhere to the principle of days on/off. A training program is also about accustoming yourself to the routine, which you want to keep consistent.

If you have come into this program with a running base (such as the one you gain by using the beginner's program in the book), you probably have a solid aerobic (heart and lungs) foundation of endurance. You may find yourself feeling that your lung power isn't tested. However, aerobic conditioning occurs sooner than lower body fitness. The training program is also for your legs to adapt to the impact. This goes not only for the muscles, but also for the connective ligaments, tendons, joints, etc. Understanding and respecting the physical adaptation mechanism of your entire body will help ensure a most successful outcome.

WARM UP, COOL DOWN, STRETCH

Warm up by working your way into the run by running five to ten minutes at a very easy pace. You can stretch after you are warmed up, or wait until after the run to stretch (but always stretch after the run). You can cool down by ending your run with several minutes of walking. Make sure to rehydrate and refuel sufficiently before, during, and after your long runs. After the long runs, a cool, or even cold, ten minute bath full enough to cover your legs aids recovery, as does putting your feet up.

THE FUNCTION OF RECOVERY

Remember the principle of hard/easy? That means that for each day of intense activity, you need time off to recover. Obviously, the days off from running built into this program give your body time to recover. But in order to

Begin and end each run, and race, with a careful warmup and cooldown. This helps you to avoid soreness or injury (right).

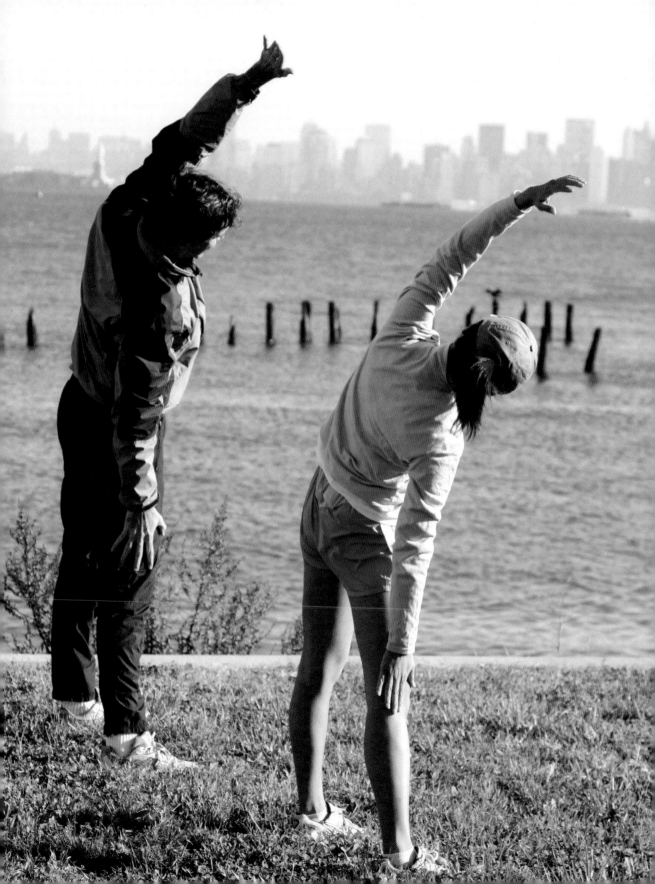

appreciate the importance of recovery, it helps to understand the physiology of training. Technically, it's not training that builds your body. Training actually breaks muscle down. Muscle is rebuilt, and thus you are strengthened, during recovery. So recovery is equally important to training. The recovery/rebuilding process also goes hand in hand with sufficient rest, good diet, and other positive lifestyle habits.

What constitutes a rest day? You don't have to cease all activity on your days off from running. On my days off running, I did my housecleaning chores, or went for a walk. Also, keep in mind that it isn't a rest day just because you don't run. If your days off running are extremely stressful for reasons not related to running, you should consider taking yet another rest day. Stress is stress, and all stress has an impact on your training. I wish I had taken more rest. I was so driven; I trained relentlessly. That's why I continually caution you *not* to make the same mistake.

The purpose of the built-in "recovery" (easy) week at week five and again at week ten is to take a physical and mental break and regroup. When you do, the recovery week, you'll say, "This is too easy. I can do this." That's good for your confidence as well.

THE 10:1 RUN/WALK PROGRAM

In the section on training, I discuss the benefits of a walk/run approach to training. John Stanton, founder of Canada's Running Room clinics, has trained thousands of people, most with no exercise background, who have successfully used his run/walk method to complete a marathon.

In his 10:1 training program, you simply run for ten minutes and walk for one. Note that your walk should be brisk, because it serves as "active rest." That keeps the heart rate moderately elevated, which helps alleviate the chemical reaction that contributes to sore and stiff muscles. Stanton refers to this as the "I'm late to an appointment" type of walking. It's quick, but still comfortable.

Stanton says that another function of the walk breaks is that they are a good time for a form check. Make sure you are running tall, with your hips slightly forward, with relaxed shoulders and arm movements (for more on running form, see that section in Chapter 6). Occupy your time during the walk by doing that form check and having a sip of water, and then it's time to get running again. "The little rest break can rejuvenate you," he says. Then, every fourth walk break (about every forty-five minutes), Stanton recommends some nutrition (e.g., gel or sports bar) to keep your blood sugar up. Again, you should test this, or any routine, in training before doing it in the race.

PRACTICING IN OTHER RACES

Practice makes perfect, as the saying goes. As I explained previously, while there may not be perfect preparation, there can be thorough preparation. In that vein, I strongly recommend that you run at least one, preferably two, other races at intermediate distances before your marathon. If you have never pinned on a race number, or used a computer chip on your shoe (if that technology applies to the

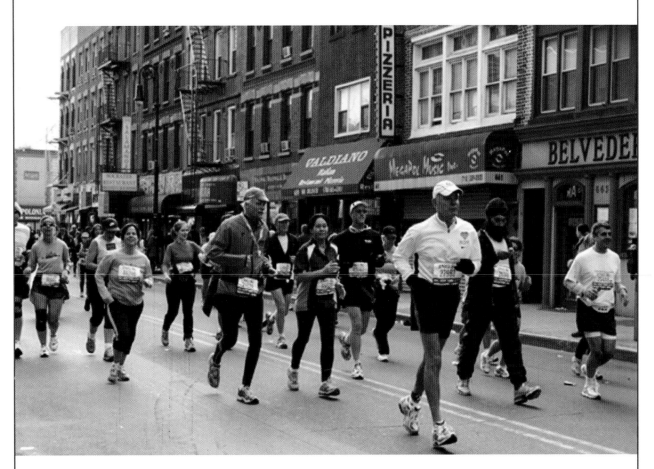

Consider taking walking breaks during the marathon. Practice them first in training.

race you enter, see the chip in the photo of shoes in Chapter 10), needed a port-a-potty, lined up and shared the road with other runners, or felt the butterflies in your stomach, it is important to have these experiences. Also, a finishing time in other races can help you calculate what you might expect to do in the marathon. It doesn't have to be a big, crowded race like the actual marathon might be. It can be a small race in the neighborhood—just as long as you get used to the ritual and routine.

Here are some practice tips for making your race experience go smoothly. They also apply to the marathon:

Register Early

To save time and money and to ensure a spot, pre-register for your race. Most races allow post-entry (signing up on site, before the event, which is slightly more expensive). If you plan to post-enter, allow extra time, and bring cash or a check. On race day, make sure to allow time to pick up your packet (race number, safety pins, T-shirt, and other goodies).

Study the Application, and the Web Site, If One Is Available

Review all the details of the race, such as course description, location of water stations, toilets, baggage area (if applicable), etc.

Plan Ahead

Pack your bag ahead of time, with your race gear, change of clothes, snacks, water, and any "emergency items" (Band-Aids, toilet paper, cell phone, money).

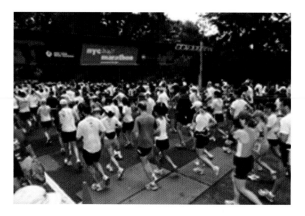

Practice races teach you to negotiate a crowded start. (Notice the rubber mat, which works in conjunction with a computer timing chip attached to the runners' shoes.)

Arrive Early, but Not Too Early

Make sure you know how to get to the race start, if it is in a new destination. Often races, and parking, can be crowded. On the other hand, don't get to the race so early you spend all your energy keeping warm (or cool) and waiting in line for the toilets.

Drink and Eat What Is Familiar

Drink enough water before the start (see Chapter 12). Be aware that nervous energy often has you looking for the toilet. That's natural and a familiar ritual for runners. Avoid caffeinated beverages if possible, which act as diuretics and can cause dehydration, or keep them to a minimum.

Don't Suddenly Stop Once You Cross the Finish Line

Make sure to cool down by continuing to move, such as by walking. Change into dry clothes, and stretch to stay loose and avoid post-race muscle stiffness. Drink water and have a snack or meal within thirty to sixty minutes, to most efficiently refuel muscles.

Recover

A race is a significant physical and mental effort. Make sure you use your days off in the training program to fully recover. You may not feel sore right away, but later. A common phenomenon is called DOMS, delayed onset muscle soreness. This is caused by small tears in the muscle fibers and should subside within several days. To assist recovery, you can walk or do other gentle physical activity to increase circulation, and continue to stretch.

10K (6.2 MILES)

By week five, your training will have prepared you to run this distance You can still walk during the race if you feel the need, or you may want to practice the 10:1 run/walk program. These days, many races at all distances are populated by walkers, some of whom walk the entire way, so you won't be alone. Some aspiring marathoners wonder about a 5K, which is actually the most popular of all race distances. But that's too short for an aspiring marathoner. A 10K is a good blend of effort—short enough not to extend you beyond what you've trained for to that point, but long enough to get the feeling of being out there for a while. If this is the first race you've ever run, take it especially easy for the first half, so you can be assured of having a strong finish and thus a good experience. You don't want to hurt too much, or "die" (radically slow down) before the end. You want to cross the finish line with positive thoughts about racing. If after a conservatively paced first half you are feeling good, however, you can pick up the pace for the rest of the way. If you want to push it (i.e., extend your effort), wait until the last mile to do so.

HALF MARATHON

Not only is this distance a good test for the marathon, it is also good for those who feel they were just getting going in a 10K and are physically and mentally primed to go further. A half marathon is a good test of your endurance, without the physical punishment of going the full 26.2 miles. More so even than the 10K, it will teach you about patience, pacing, and how to negotiate a wider range of physical and emotional cycles. Your guideline for how you approach this race should be based on your training. You should pace yourself similarly to your long training runs. If you are taking walking breaks in training, do so in this race. Make sure you have practiced drinking (and taking in nutrition) during your training runs, since you will want to do so in this race.

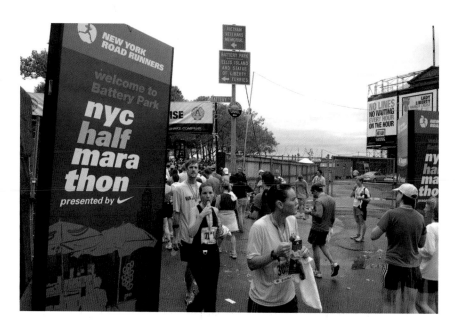

Running a half marathon is an important rehearsal for the full 26.2-mile event.

A GOOD FORMULA

While I emphasize that you should not run your first marathon for time, it is helpful (and fun!) to have a general benchmark, at least to assist you in where to line up at the start and how to pace yourself. Noted English coach Frank Horwill has come up with what he calls his Five Pace Theory of training for the marathon, detailed in an article on the Serpentine Running Club Web site His numbers were calculated for elite runners; however, I feel his 10K and half marathon prediction formulas also seem sound for novices.

You can roughly guess your running time for the marathon by calculating five times your 10K time minus ten minutes. You can predict a marathon time by multiplying your half marathon times two, plus six and a half minutes.

HOW TO READ THE CHARTS

The weeks go from top to bottom and include the mileage for four days, with the total for the week in the last column. You can plan your running days according to your own schedule and the way you are feeling. However, do not run four days in a row. Spread the days out to allow for recovery. The longer or harder the run, the greater the need is to follow it up with time off.

It's a good idea to gain experience by running one, preferably two, shorter races. If you want to do a 10K, the best time to schedule it is during the first cutback, in week five. For a half marathon, it would be week ten. I recommend doing both races.

16-WEEK BEGINNING MARATHON PROGRAM

Week					Total
1	3	3	3	5	14
2	3	4	4	5	16
3	4	4	4	6	18
4	4	4	4	8	20
5	3	3	3	6	15 (cut back week, 10K race)
6	4	5	4	9	22
7	5	5	4	10	24
8	5	6	4	12	27
9	5	6	5	13	29
10	4	4	4	10	22 (cut back week, Half Mar. race)
11	6	6	5	14	31
12	6	6	5	16	33
13	6	7	6	18	37
14	6	8	6	20	40
15	4	5	4	13	26
16	3	4	3	10	20

You can choose from:

Choice A: run Monday, Wednesday, Friday, long run on Saturday.

Choice B: run Tuesday, Wednesday, Friday, long run on Sunday.

Choice C: run Monday, Wednesday, Thursday, long run on Saturday.

You can mix up the training days each week, just as long as you take time off the day after the long run.

6

Running Basics

PACING YOURSELF—HOW FAST SHOULD YOU TRAIN?

Your marathon goal has been firmly established: The most important thing is going the distance. And while you won't be watching the clock with a goal time in mind, you still need to be aware of how to establish the proper training pace, which you will later attempt to maintain during your marathon. The proper pace keeps you both in your comfort zone and, most importantly, from going too fast and undermining your efforts.

The most accurate way to gauge the proper pace is the scientific way, by using your heart rate and a mathematical formula. The first step is to determine your maximum heart rate (MHR). This is the maximum level of your heart's ability to pump blood and deliver it to your body. From there, you can derive the optimum heart rate for training.

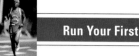

The traditional formula for determining MHR is the maximum of 220 minus your age. But the aforementioned Frank Horwill, founder of the British Milers Club way back in 1963 and advisor to the Serpentine Running Club, has a heart rate formula I feel is more accurate than the old standard calculation. He explains, "The old method was to take 220 beats per minute as maximum, and then to subtract from that figure one's age. So, a twenty-five-year-old female would use this formula: 220 minus 25 = 195 bpm (beats per minute) maximum." Horwill feels you can get even closer. He quotes recent research that suggests a more accurate estimation: 209 beats per minute maximum minus 0.7 for every year of age. So, the new equation for the twenty-five-year-old woman

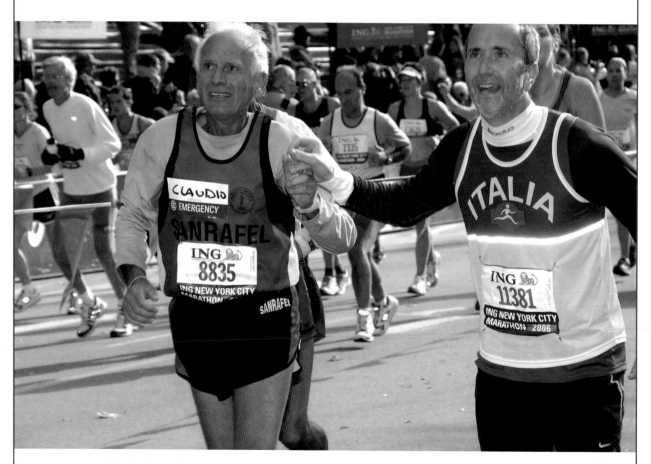

Pacing is crucial. A member of the worldwide Achilles Track Club for the disabled, and his guide, are pictured here.

would be: 209 minus 25×0.7 (17.5) = 191.5 bpm. (Note this is slightly lower than the old calculation.)

Howell calculates the figures for males somewhat differently, using 214 bpm minus 0.8 for every year of age. So for a twenty-five-year-old male, the formula is: 214 minus 25×0.8 (20) = 194 bpm. (Note that the old formula is more accurate for men than women.)

This is a very general guideline. Individual MHR may vary by as much as 30 to 40 beats up or down from any general mathematical formula, depending on the person. However, with medical approval and no underlying health issues, you can determine your MHR with a physical test if you wish. Usually MHR is determined by testing on a treadmill or bike, but a less intense method is a sub-maximal heart rate test. This does not require an all-out effort and can be determined by trainers or sports medicine personnel at fitness centers or gyms. In fact, this test is often administered or even required before you join a health club, although you may be able to schedule one without joining.

There are self-tests for reaching maximal heart rate, such as sprinting a given distance or on an uphill a number of times; when you have reached exhaustion, then take your pulse. However, I think this can be difficult for a beginner not used to hard running and may result in failure to achieve an accurate result. Also, it can be physically risky to extend yourself in these tests when you are not conditioned to do so.

Once you have your calculations, you can use a heart rate monitor or measure your pulse manually. To measure by hand, put your index and third finger (do not use your thumb, which is not as sensitive as your other fingers) and place them on your throat or the inside of your wrist until you feel the strongest beat. Count to six and multiply by ten for the most accurate value, as your heart rate rapidly slows during a longer count.

Once you have calculated your MHR, you can proceed to train by these guidelines:

Training for "heart health" means working at 60 to 70 percent of MHR. Anything above 80 percent is anaerobic, or without oxygen. This occurs during serious, intense running, such as intervals (measured bursts of speed followed by recovery) or other forms of speed training.

Seventy to eighty percent of MHR is the aerobic zone. Most of your training for the marathon will be in this zone. Also known as the endurance-building zone, this training pace should feel as if you are on "cruise control." In this zone, you should be comfortable enough when running that you can pass the "talk test." That is, you can carry on a conversation while running without feeling out of breath.

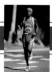
To give you an idea of how your conditioning is progressing and ultimately to chart your recovery from more strenuous efforts, you will also want to establish your resting heart rate. This is best calculated by measuring your pulse at the same time each day, such as right before getting out of bed in the morning. You will notice that as you get fitter, this number goes down, as your heart (your largest muscle) becomes stronger and more efficient at supplying blood to your body.

As you become fitter, your recovery rate will also improve; that is, the time it takes for your pulse rate to return to normal after effort. Once you become familiar with your various heart rates, you can use this information to gauge your fitness and recovery. It's a good idea to keep track of heart rates in your training diary.

OTHER METHODS FOR MEASURING YOUR EFFORTS

Some experts recommend using what's called perceived exertion, or how your body feels, to determine your effort. This is as simple as rating effort from numbers 1 to 10 (with 10 being the greatest effort). While this is obviously less complicated, it is a measure that is based entirely on subjectivity. Under the best of circumstances, this is a risky gauge of effort. Without significant experience, it is almost impossible to judge the value of perceived effort. Also, as a beginner with an ambitious goal like the marathon, it is important not to risk either under- or overestimating your effort—both of which can greatly compromise your desired result.

On the other end of the spectrum, once you have your heart rate values, there is an even more scientific and accurate way to keep track of proper pace. That's with a heart rate monitor (HRM). A heart rate monitor is a lightweight device consisting of a belt that is wrapped around the chest, which acts as a transmission device for the receiver, a wristwatch. The belt relays your heart rate to the watch, giving you immediate feedback.

For most of my career, I never scientifically measured my heart rate. But when heart rate monitors gained popularity, I finally tried one. Even after all my years of running, I learned a lot. It proved to me that even the most experienced runner can fall victim to the inaccuracy of "perceived exertion." With the heart rate monitor, I discovered that I was regularly overdoing it. My runs on my easy days were too fast, and I was also not allowing enough recovery time between intense efforts. (For information on purchasing a heart rate monitor, see Chapter 10.)

HOW FAR HAVE YOU RUN?

A useful Web site for the running community can let you know how far you've run—anywhere in the world. You can check out your routes at home, or chart courses for destinations you're planning to visit. Simply go to Googleearth.com, where you can download a free program that has a satellite map, and put in any address worldwide. This mapping tool allows you to measure your course to within .01 of miles.

RUNNING FORM

Everyone knows how to run, right? You did it as a child, so it should seem natural to you as an adult. Although you might think so, chances are that many years have transpired since you experienced this "natural" activity, so you may feel out of sync or uncoordinated when you first begin to run. The beauty of running is that although it may have lain dormant, it is not forgotten. Your body does have a natural gait, and as you gain experience, you will become more efficient at it. That being said, running doesn't feel comfortable in the beginning for some people. Or some people feel insecure about it. I coached one woman who told me she had to learn because, she said, "I never ran in my entire life." Her lesson was casual. She had someone go out and run with her around the block a few times to show her the ropes and check her form.

Contrary to a common myth, while there are general guidelines, there is no exactly "right" way to run. I grew up with running, so I thought I knew what runners looked like. But I've been watching races from the sidelines for years, and I am amazed by the many ways people move forward. Some shuffle, barely lifting their legs or their bodies, but they move quickly. Some have a long or bouncing stride; some take short, choppy steps. Some barely pump their arms. When the argument used to come up, and people wanted to prove that there was no exact form for running well, they always brought up Bill Rodgers. Bill has an odd habit of swinging one of his arms out to the side on every stride, but that certainly didn't affect his ability to win four Boston and four New York City Marathons.

I don't recommend you attempt to drastically alter your form. You have to let yourself run more or less naturally. I know this from personal experience. In the height of my career, I had a new coach from Eastern Europe who told me that I'd run faster if I changed my stride. I worked hard to comply, and while I may have been running technically more "correct," the effort it took slowed my times. In fact, it sabotaged my entire season.

While you can practice good running form, it is very hard to do so consciously. Children are a good illustration. They don't deliberately think about their form, but good young runners move very efficiently and economically. The slower ones are not as technically sound. There are reasons you don't want your arms and legs moving all over the place. Solid running form not only helps you run better (farther and faster), but helps you to avoid injuries as well.

While you shouldn't tinker with your running form too much, there are good habits you can establish. Below are some tips for good running form. If you want to check your form, run on a treadmill in front of a mirror, or glance at your reflection when running by storefront windows.

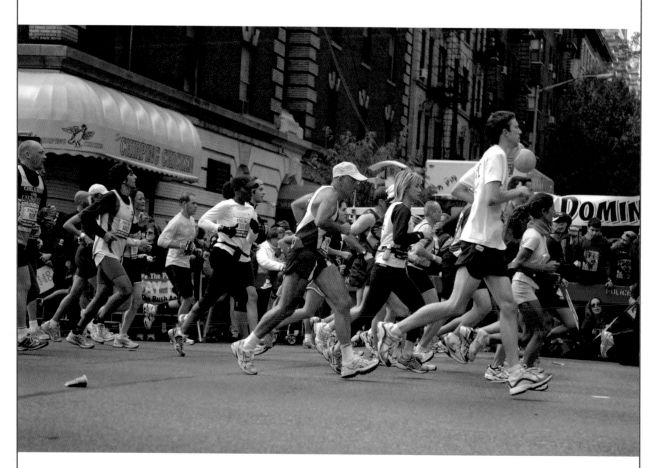

Run relaxed with upright posture, hands loosely cupped and shoulders dropped.

Don't Plod

You can hear some runners by the sound of their pounding feet. Try to keep your foot plant light and quick.

Don't Over-Stride or Under-Stride

A proper stride length should feel natural; over-or under-doing it feels awkward and can contribute to injury.

Don't Run up on Your Toes

I notice this habit especially among some women. Instead, the heel naturally strikes the ground before you roll onto the ball of your foot.

Watch Your Arm Carriage

Hold your arms at the midpoint of your body and swing them pendulum fashion, back to front, not side to side. Keep your hands loosely cupped, neither clenched nor flopping. Your arms naturally cross the midpoint of your chest as they swing forward.

Maintain Good Posture

Stand erect (but not stiff), and take care not to slouch over, particularly if you begin to fatigue.

RELAXATION AND BREATHING

Running with a relaxed effort is most efficient. Focus on keeping your face, neck, and shoulders loose, as opposed to gritting your teeth and clenching your fists. Tension requires energy, and that detracts from your running. If you watch good runners (a good idea, by the way), you notice that their faces look very natural, even loose (although in a race or effort, they may have a more intense look of concentration). Many beginners ask if they should breathe only through their nose, or only through their mouth. Like everything else about running form, breathe naturally, which is through both your nose and mouth. Like form, breathing comes in all styles. Some people make very little noise when they run; some huff and puff. Do what feels right for you. Remember though, that while it's okay to be a heavy breather—to expel breath with effort—don't breathe shallowly or fast. This causes you to suck in more air than you expel, which is a major cause of cramps or side stitches.

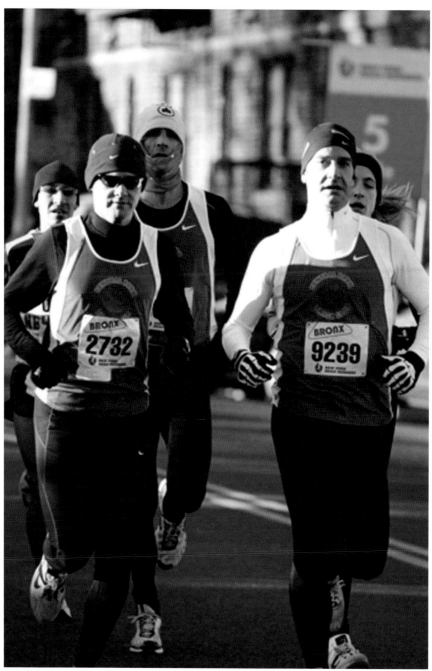

Do a "form check" periodically. Make sure you are running loose and relaxed, particularly your upper body.

(This painful problem can also arise from eating too close to the time you run.) If this tends to happen to you at any point, or to avoid it in the first place, focus on consciously expelling air through your teeth and mouth about every fourth breath. This also helps calm you down, as nervousness can result in shallow or rapid breathing. If you do get a cramp or a stitch, try bending over and applying pressure to the spot where it originates, or raise your arm over your head to stretch it out.

No question about it, standing on the starting line of a race and waiting to begin is nerve-wracking. To help get rid of excess tension and to remain relaxed, try taking some precautionary deep breathes to keep you calm, and shake out your arms and legs and roll your head while focusing on dropping your shoulders.

PRACTICING ON THE RUN

In addition to getting your body acclimated to the effort of pounding out the miles, you will want to practice other aspects of the marathon. Particularly during your long runs, get used to drinking and consuming whatever nutrition you will use in the race, such as gels or bars. I always used sports drinks. For my training runs, I either put them out along the course before the run, or Jack brought them to me in the car. I often used the technique many runners do the day before a long run. I drove the course and planted some sports drink bottles, usually behind trees or other landmarks. Sometimes, I ran with a drink belt around my waist, which you can purchase in a running specialty store. The best one I have found has several small bottles. Just make sure to fasten it so it doesn't bounce when you run (for more on drink devices, see Chapter 10).

A call to the toilet is a sensitive issue, but one you cannot ignore. You need to know what to expect when you run the marathon. I was never particularly concerned during training if "nature called," but I was always more careful for the race. One of my most dramatic race stories is also my most awkward. I was in the lead of the London Marathon when I got an attack of diarrhea. (This happened again, in New York.) In my mind, there was no question: I had to keep running, despite the shock of onlookers and worse, the television cameras broadcasting the event to millions of people. If I had stopped the race, for any reason, I would have lost. It was not a pleasant experience, but winning those races was. Nevertheless, it was a problem I had to learn to solve.

As nutritionist Nancy Clark confirms, this problem is more common than people realize, particularly among beginners. I get questions about it often at clinics and autograph signings. And what's more, on even the most well equipped race course or training loop, it seems a bathroom is never there when you need it. I had the problem in training as well, so that's where I learned to conquer it. I resorted to taking an over-the-counter anti-diarrhea medicine, and I also watched my diet leading up to the run (see Nutrition, Chapter 12). I took these steps for any run over an hour. It solved the problem for me. If you experience any problems, training runs are a good time to learn how to cope. Again, if you are considering making any adjustments, practice them first in training.

7

Training Extras

Cross training, the practice of doing a variety of exercise activities or sports, is a great habit for general fitness. It also comes in handy to protect runners from the repetitive motion and pounding we endure in our sport, the result of which can be injury or burnout. It's another major topic of inquiry when I do running clinics. These days, many more recreational runners (and marathoners) use cross training on a regular basis. They do it to protect themselves, but to get a good workout. I think this applies to us as we get older and don't handle the pounding as well. With cross training, we can minimize the risk without sacrificing the conditioning.

Technically, you will not use cross training during your first marathon preparation (it is not built into the training program), but it can come in very handy if you need it. It is also important to consider for your marathon recovery and for keeping fit post-marathon. To this end, it's a good idea to plan ahead and have experience in the exercise you choose (e.g., learn the technique), and locate a facility, if you need one.

Even though I have great faith in the marathon program I prescribe in this book, it's risky to guarantee anyone could make it through four months of training, like clockwork, without some sort of glitch. If you get sore, or slightly injured, or if the weather, or life, prevents you from getting in your run, cross training can be there for you to maintain your basic fitness. (If you do have to take off a week or more from the program, even with cross training, you need to start back up where you left off. So, if you get hurt in week ten, don't start up again at week eleven or twelve. Go back to week ten first.)

For now, days off in the program mean no running. You need to recover between efforts. However, that doesn't mean you should be restricted to no activity at all. If you want to take a walk, or your child asks you to play basketball, it certainly doesn't hurt to engage in these activities. Don't say no to playing with your kids just because of your marathon training.

I made successful use of cross training in my own career. When I hurt my knee or foot, I was able to rest those injured areas and still get an aerobic workout, either by running in a pool with a floatation device, or using a cross-country ski machine or stationary bike. There are even stories of those marathoners forced to resort to a more long-term program of cross training who still maintain the fitness to run their marathon. If for any reason you feel you shouldn't run, try to maintain your program with another fitness activity. If possible, choose those activities that are most similar to running—such as water running or the elliptical machine. I get a good workout on a cross-country ski machine, but that's because growing up in Norway, I know how to ski. However, anything that gets your heart rate going can be effective.

Obviously, conventional sports such as biking, basketball, soccer, tennis, and cross-country skiing all fall into the category of cross training. There are many popular alternative activities you might enjoy that benefit your fitness and also develop strength, balance, and flexibility. While marathon training is your current emphasis, you might want to try them eventually.

There are many more contemporary forms of exercise and fitness that have gained popularity since I started running. Pilates and yoga are good for runners because they focus on core strength, posture, balance, and flexibility. I was once convinced to try a yoga class by a reporter when I was in Kansas City for a race promotion. I was like an elephant in a glass house, although I can certainly see the benefits of yoga, and there are many popular varieties.

I hope that after doing the marathon, you will have had a good experience getting in shape. You'll want to maintain your fitness, and weight loss, if that was a desired by-product of your training. Maybe you won't keep up running as many miles, but you can use cross training to fill out your fitness schedule.

MASSAGE

There are many benefits of massage, both physical and mental. Massage relaxes sore or tight muscles, which can both speed recovery and help prevent injury. Massage increases the blood's ability to carry oxygen, while facilitating a gentle stretch to muscles and surrounding tissues. Massage is a reward for your hard work. I regularly had various types of massage during my career, as many serious athletes do. But these days, every level of runner takes advantage of massage. Much of what I had was very deep tissue work, which can be quite painful but yields good results. You may feel it too extreme or unnecessary in your case. While massage can be relaxing and pleasurable, you may experience

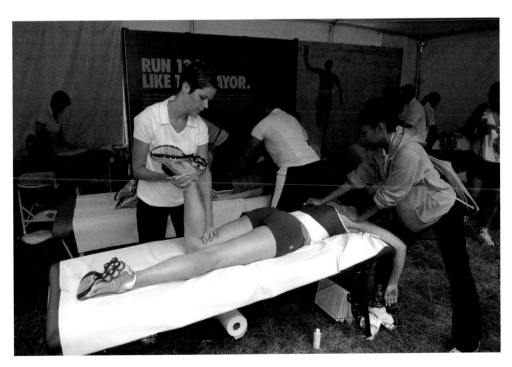

Take advantage of the relaxing and therapeutic benefits of massage, especially after your long runs.

some soreness or pain when a therapist works on tight muscles even if you don't opt for the deep tissue variety. You should communicate with the therapist and explain your training and what you want from the massage. Most therapists will ask, but make sure you express if it is too painful, or conversely, if it is not deep enough. Look for a certified massage therapist who specializes in sports massage, specifically one who treats runners, if possible. To find a good massage therapist, ask friends, or check throughout the running community via a club or a running store. You should schedule your massage for one of your days off running if possible. Also, make sure you hydrate well after your message.

Although free massage by professionals is offered after many races, the latest thinking is that it is important to wait at least two hours after a half marathon or longer event. In shorter efforts, you should be completely cooled down before receiving a massage.

While a professional massage is a treat, you don't have to go that route to experience some of the benefits. You can try partner massage, or even self-massage. Regular, light self-massage after workouts can address key areas, or you can simply start from the bottom up. Soak your feet first in warm, sudsy water. Rub the heel area, using your thumbs to apply various levels of pressure, up to fifteen seconds at a time for pressure point work (pushing into one area with your thumbs). Sit in a chair and massage your Achilles tendons and your calves. Use your palms or fingers to apply friction to the front and back of the thighs, and sit or lie on a tennis ball or similar item for pressure point work on any area of the hips, buttocks, or lower back. Also, don't forget to give a rub to the back of your neck and shoulders. In addition to using your hands, you might want to try a massage stick, which comes in various shapes and styles.

While you or a partner can give special attention to massaging problem areas, if you have severe or lasting muscle or joint pain, it is best to avoid massaging the area and to see a doctor.

From the start, my sister-in-law Wenche was well prepared to run her first marathon. Her attitude going into the race was sensible. She said, "I just want to finish, and I want to feel good about it." Of course she was nervous, but her goal was the right one. Particularly because it was New York, she was determined to get the most out of the race.

WENCHE ANDERSEN: I always said that if I ran a marathon, it would be New York, because of Grete. She's such a good friend, and she inspires me. For years, I watched her run the race, and I thought, "Sometime in my life, I want to do that." I had hoped to do it before I turned 50, but I ended up doing it at 52, because I had pain in my feet for a couple of years. I had to put off running. But Grete said to me, "You don't have to run all the time. You can walk and run." And that's what I did, in training and in the race.

I had always been working out, in the gym, doing spinning and lifting weights. I started running in July, four months before the marathon. The training went the way I thought it would. No surprises. No problems. Even though I knew I wanted to run the race with my husband, I did all the training by myself. It wasn't hard for me. I liked it that way.

I asked for Grete's advice, especially since it was my first time. She emphasized, "You have to take it slowly, not be in a hurry." I was very lucky I had my husband (Grete's brother Arild) and my brother-in-law (Grete's brother Jan) to run the race with me.

The race was great, and I was really excited to do it. After three hours though, my right foot started to hurt. Arild and Jan kept encouraging me, and people everywhere were saying, "You're looking great." That really helped. And, too, Grete had been my inspiration to run, so I wanted to have a great race for her.

I held back, because Grete had warned me not to let others pull me along, which turned out to be the most important advice I got. Arild and Jan kept trying to push me to go faster, but I stuck to what Grete said: run/walk. I'd run for three miles, and then do a 100-meter walk.

The experience was even better than I imagined, because everything was so well organized, and the people were fantastic. That support really helps. In fact, I'm doing the race again this year. Although I hope I can run what I did last year, I'm not doing it for time, but to have the same experience again.

Norwegians love Grete. She's a great person. She especially appeals to ordinary people, because she's got both feet on the ground. Having run New York, I have an even greater appreciation for what she did.

HOW AND WHY TO KEEP A DIARY

Keeping track of your training is great race preparation. A diary functions as a coach, psychiatrist, and conscience. By making a personal study of your experience—what you do and how you feel—you can keep on track for a successful race. I believe that because you are investing so greatly in your marathon endeavor, you owe it to yourself to do everything you can, including keeping a diary. And, too, don't forget, half the journey to the starting line is getting there. You want to value the training as a process in and of itself. A diary helps you to do that.

I kept training diaries for nearly twenty years. I used them often for reference, especially to get myself psyched up, for inspiration, or to study the reasons when things went either right or wrong. The diary is a more objective account of your training, as opposed to simply counting on your memory. It's difficult to keep track of your many weeks of training from memory. A diary can also be a great motivator. In keeping a daily record, no one wants to have to write, "Didn't run today; didn't feel like it." A diary can give you confidence. If you experience the normal doubts leading up to the marathon, you can page through your diary to see the work you've put in. It can also be very entertaining or inspiring to look back at the diary as a memento of your marathon experience.

You will be amazed as you look over your diary, using it as a training tool, which you should do throughout the weeks leading up to the race, to see what a revelation it can be. Study the stressful weeks, and attempt to avoid them. Study the successful weeks, and attempt to duplicate them.

To keep up with your diary, make it convenient. Use a published runner's log, calendar, notebook, the computer—whatever you like. There are also several online running diaries. (Both CoolRunning.com and MarathonGuide.com have one for members that is free of charge.) When keeping your diary, record the number of miles, the type of course, including the road surface, terrain (e.g., hilly, flat) or treadmill settings, and the weather, and include a general notation on how you felt. Whether you feel great, or experience any excessive fatigue, aches, or soreness, it is important to keep track. The greater the detail, the more useful the diary will be.

STRETCHING AND STRENGTHENING

I probably should have stretched more in my competitive days, although I was part of a generation of runners that was not as enlightened as I later became. In the 1990s, I received the assistance of my sports massage and sports injury therapist, Gerard Hartmann of Ireland. Gerard, also a seven-time Irish national triathlon champion, has treated dozens of Olympians and is considered an expert worldwide.

Running is a restrictive and repetitive movement. The constant pounding of the activity is also hard on the body. That's why it is important to stretch and strengthen certain muscles to help create a physical balance. Stretching ensures flexibility, and strengthening addresses the muscles not developed through running, such as those of the core and upper body.

Begin with stretching. These simple exercises should take you no more than ten to fifteen minutes and can be done anywhere. I prefer to stretch post-run, even after a shower, when my muscles are loose and I've recovered from my workout.

I recommend a system called active-isolated stretching. In this system, the muscles are held in the safest and most relaxed anatomical positions, isolated with localized movements for maximum flexibility, and stretched for a brief time period (five to eight seconds), with each exercise repeated five to eight times. Holding the stretch for brief periods stimulates blood and oxygen flow to the muscle and encourages it to lengthen (which promotes flexibility). Holding the stretch for a longer time period causes the muscle to contract to protect itself, resulting in an effort to return to its natural state. Only a relaxed muscle can be stretched. When stretching, never bounce, use jerky movements, or stretch too quickly or to the point of pain. Although traditionally done after warming up, you can also stretch to warm up, if you do so carefully.

Hamstring Stretch

Keep your non-stretched leg straight out and on the ground. Keeping your other leg straight, use the strength of your quadriceps (front thigh muscle) to pull your leg up as far as you can. Then, take a rope or towel and extend it over the bottom of your left foot. Hold the two ends and gently pull your leg toward your head until you feel the stretch. Concentrate on relaxing the hamstring muscle. Release to the nonstretch position. After repeating the exercise five to eight times, switch legs and repeat. You should feel the stretch only in the back of your thigh. Take care not to stretch to the point you feel it in the back of your knee.

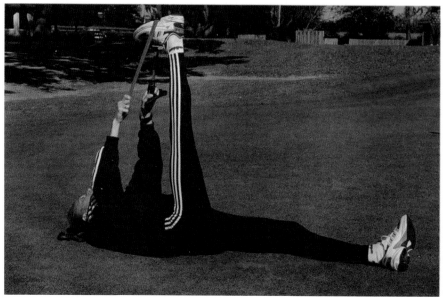

Hamstring Stretch

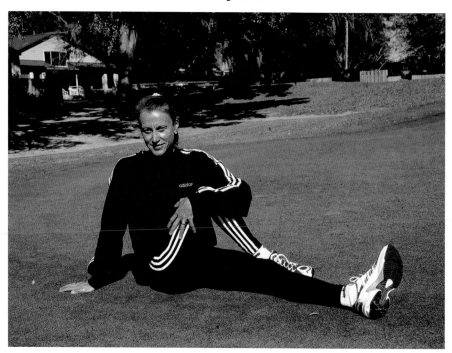

Gluteal Muscle Stretch

Gluteal Muscle Stretches

Extend the left leg and bend the right. Cross your right foot over the straight leg and put it next to the outside of the left knee. Wrap your left arm around the outside of the right knee. Twist the top of your body to the right, while gently pulling the knee toward your chest. You should feel the stretch in the right buttocks muscle. Switch legs and repeat.

Quadriceps Stretch

Lie on your right side and extend your left leg. Hooking your right arm under your right knee, bring your right knee to your chest. This stabilizes the pelvis and the spine. Pull your left foot toward your buttocks with your left hand. Switch legs and repeat.

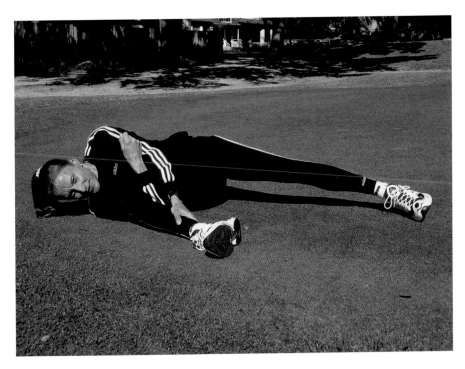

Quadriceps Stretch

Calf Stretches

Most people do this stretch standing up, but in keeping with the philosophy of the other stretches (muscle in its relaxed position), Gerard suggests doing it while sitting.

1. Sitting on the floor with your legs extended, put a rope or towel around the bottom of your right foot. Pull back on your toes until you feel the stretch in your calf. Bend the left knee if it is a more comfortable position. Switch legs and repeat.
2. Facing the wall at about arm's length put your right leg one to two feet behind the left. Keeping the right leg straight and the left knee bent, lean on the wall. Make sure your right heel is on the ground, and your back is straight. Then, slowly lean into the wall. Switch legs and repeat.
3. Do the same stretch, but bend the right knee, in order to stretch the lower calf and Achilles tendon.

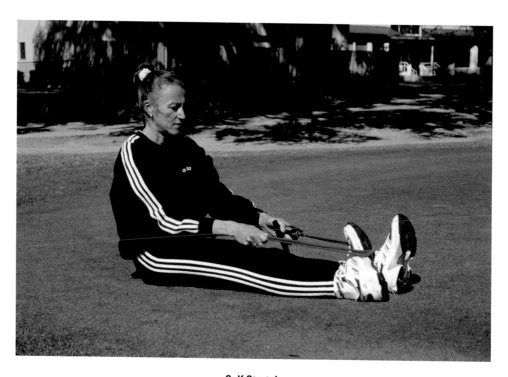

Calf Stretch

Upper body stretches are good to assist your running posture, which is particularly important as you tire over the long run.

Lateral Trunk Stretch

This stretch is good for the neck, chest, upper back, and shoulders.

1. Extend your right arm over your head and place it over your left ear. Your left arm should remain at your side.
2. Lean to your left until your left arm reaches down to the side of your left knee. Switch arms and repeat.

Triceps Stretch

This stretch, often called "scratch your back," is for flexibility at the back of the upper arm.

1. Bend your right arm so that you are able to reach your right hand down your back. With your left hand, reach over your head and grasp your right elbow. Then gently push back on the right elbow. Switch arms and repeat.

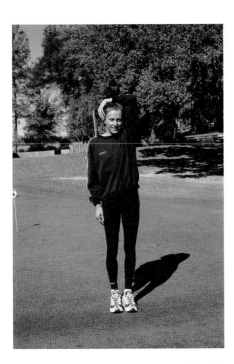 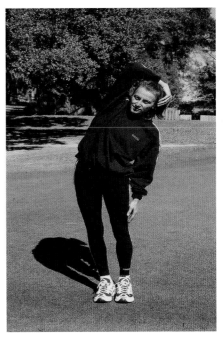

Lateral Trunk Stretch

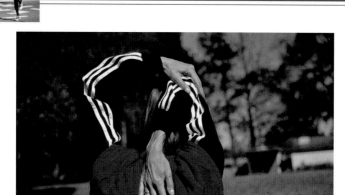

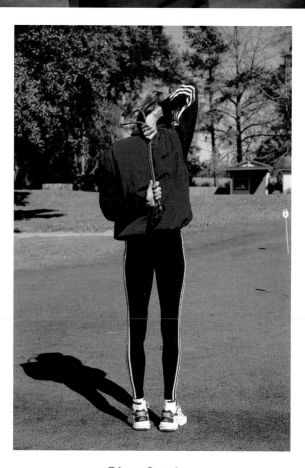

Triceps Stretch

2. If you are more limber, try this variation. Drop your right hand down your back. Bring your left hand up your back and reach toward your right hand. To assist with this stretch, drop a towel down your back and grab it with your left hand.

STRENGTHENING

Many marathoners make the mistake of conditioning only the parts of the body used for their sport. But strengthening muscles not directly addressed by running can help ensure you remain injury-free, and it can help you become a stronger runner (after all, your upper body has to go 26.2 miles as well). Basic strengthening is important, particularly as we age and experience a decrease in muscle mass and strength. Just as with stretching, these exercises will be an excellent supplement to any post-marathon running or exercise.

Crunches

Popular activities such as Pilates and gym and health club classes emphasize the importance of core strength. Many runners do not recognize the connection between exercises such as crunches and their activity. Crunches help protect the lower back. You want to strengthen the trunk flexors, which are only worked during the first 20 percent of a true sit-up. A crunch is executed by rising only to the point that you feel the muscle contract, with just the shoulders and upper back coming off the ground. Work your way up to two or three sets (fifteen to twenty crunches per set) of each type of crunch.

1. Keeping your feet flat on the floor, bend your knees and cross your hands on your chest. (It's fine to put your hands on the sides of your head, but clasping them behind your head allows you to tug, which creates strain on the neck.)
2. Raise your body straight up until your shoulders and upper back are off the floor. Do one set of fifteen to twenty of these.
3. As you rise, twist to touch your elbow to the opposite thigh. This works a different set of abdominal muscles than the first exercise. Do one set of these.
4. This is a more complex crunch, but with added benefits. With your knees bent, raise your legs in the air and cross your ankles. To up it even further, place a five- or ten-pound weight on your chest while doing the exercise.

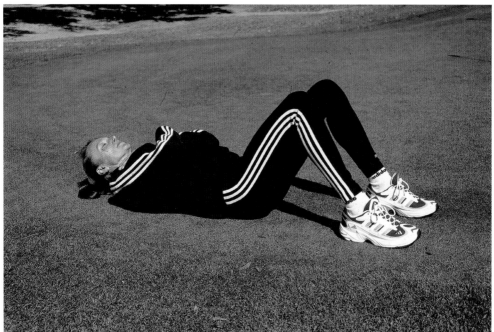

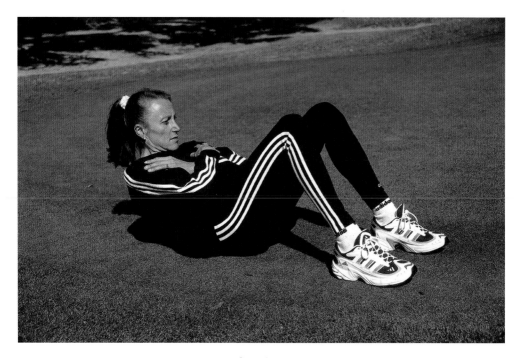

Crunches 1–2

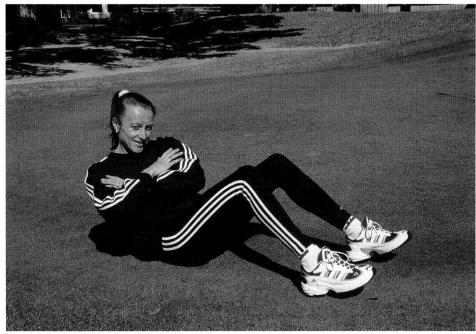

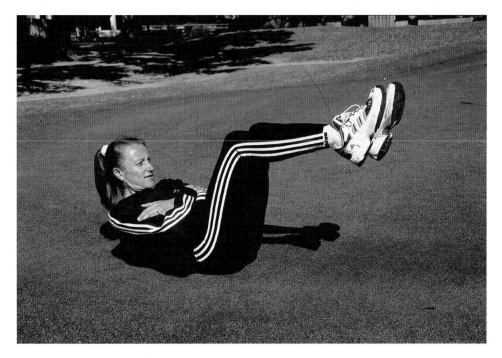

Crunches 3–4

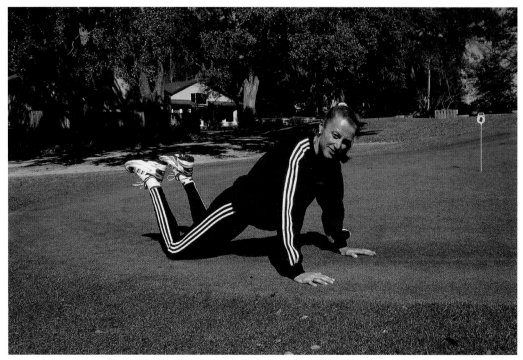

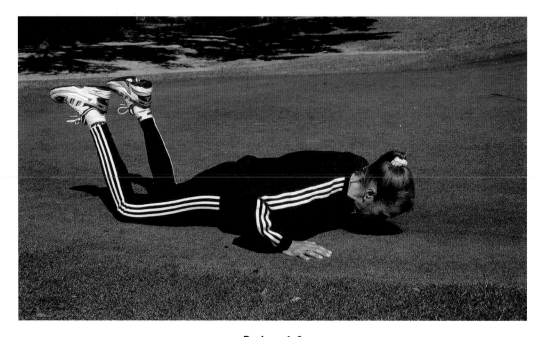

Pushups 1–2

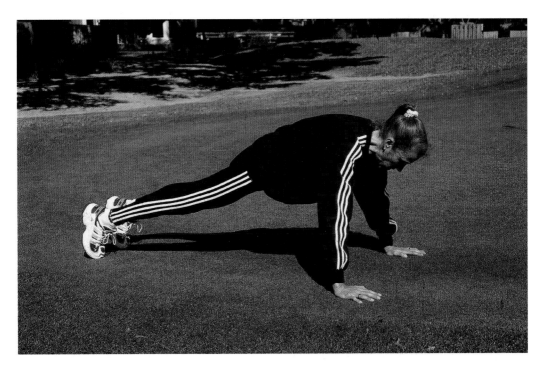

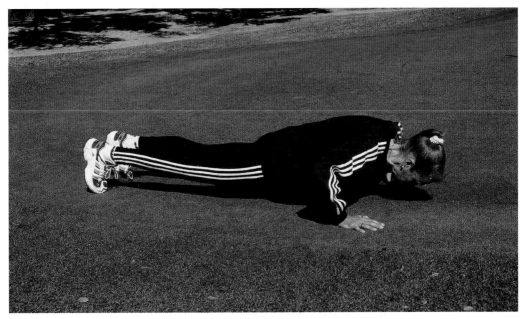

Pushups 3–4

Push-Ups

1. Since push-ups can be difficult, beginners may find it easier to start with this version, in which you do the push-ups with the knees bent and the feet in the air. Place your hands shoulder width apart.
2. Keeping your back straight (like a plank) and your palms flat on the floor, lower yourself until your chin nearly touches the floor.
3. For the standard push-up, position your body at about a forty-five-degree angle to the floor. Support your weight on your palms and toes. Do not lock your elbows; keep them slightly bent. Your feet should be placed together; your feet and hands point forward. Keep your legs, back, and neck in a straight line. (You strain your neck by looking up).
4. Lower yourself until your body is parallel to the floor. Return to the starting position.

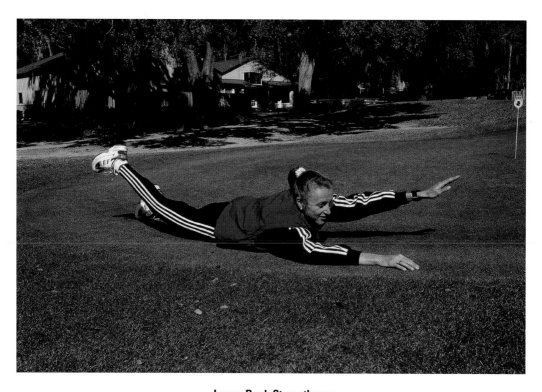

Lower Back Strengthener

Lower Back Strengthener

Lie on your stomach with your legs extended. Raise your right leg about six inches off the floor and simultaneously raise your left arm. Lift your head slightly at the same time. Hold the position for two seconds, and then switch to the other leg and arm. Start with two to three sets of ten, and build up to sets of twenty.

Heel Drops

This exercise was referred to in Chapter 7. It strengthens the Achilles tendon, helping to prevent Achilles tendonitis (or a tear of the calf muscle).

Do this exercise fairly rapidly and rhythmically. Focus on the down portion. Do not rise up high on your toes when you come back up. Do three sets of ten. By the third set, you should feel a slight burning sensation in your calves.

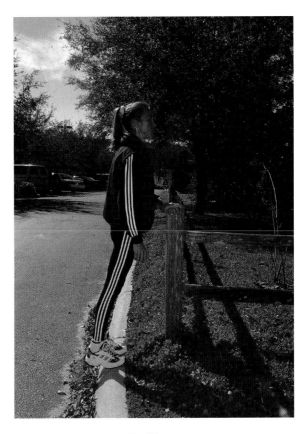

Heel Drops

8

The Running Life

FITTING IT IN

You've made the marathon commitment; now the challenge is to do the training. Often the issue is not so much *how* to do the training, but *when* to do it. After all, you can't do your homework properly if you don't have the time and energy. There are a variety of considerations for fitting your training into your lifestyle. Some are practical (e.g., where and when you work, or when family obligations are scheduled); some are physical and psychological (e.g., are you a morning, afternoon, or evening person?).

In marathon training, timing is everything. Most people I know who are preparing for the marathon (or doing any exercise, for that matter) have learned to fit their training around their work hours. I have one friend who works various shifts at a hotel. When she decided to run a marathon, she had to train at all hours. I always felt it must be tough not to have a stable routine, but she was upbeat and determined. Although I've always preferred running in the morning, even though my mind and my body were reluctant, I also had to train daily in the afternoon. I had a standing appointment to run with my brothers, so that got me out the door. The obligation to meet them was a big help with my motivation.

In addition to a partner or group, you may need to resort to other methods to ensure you get your training done. This is one of the reasons that I stressed earlier that you will need to be well organized. Plan your runs ahead of time, perhaps week by week. Check the week's weather forecast, in the event you might want to change your long-run day. Write every session in your calendar, making an appointment with yourself. Create or join a babysitting

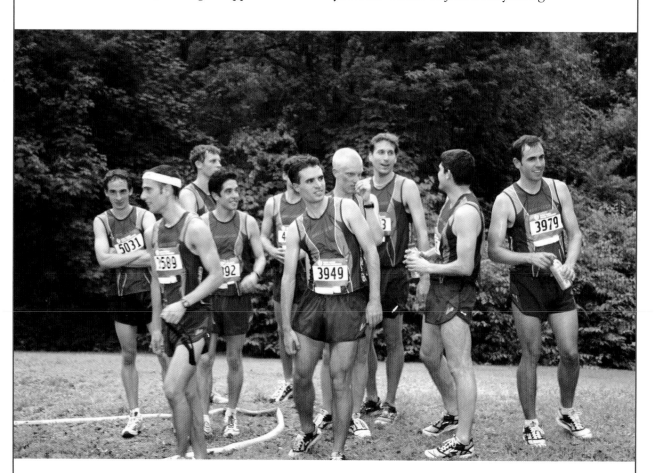

Training and racing with others strengthens your commitment and camaraderie.

co-op. I've even seen women training together while pushing their children in running strollers. Carry running gear and a change of clothes in your car, so if an opportunity to run suddenly presents itself, you're prepared to take advantage of it.

The advantage of early morning running is that you get it done and out of the way. There is little to distract you. In fact, most surveys indicate that those who work out in the morning are more likely to stick to their exercise routine than those who work out at other times of the day. But some people just can't manage mornings. They can't tolerate going from a warm bed out into the cold or, physically, their body feels too stiff, not ready to run. If you want to be a morning runner, try giving yourself thirty minutes to an hour to wake up—have some coffee, juice, or other snack, and get your blood moving by doing a few chores before heading out to run. Also, ease into the workout by starting with a slow jog. If you're reluctant to go straight out into the cold, you can warm up inside first by running in place, jumping rope, doing several sets of walking up stairs, or using other exercise equipment.

From a physiological perspective, exercise in the afternoon or early evening is most ideal. The body temperature is higher, and the muscles and joints are more flexible. However, if you are pressed for time, fall victim to scheduling conflicts, or just feel too tired, all physical advantage of an afternoon run is obviously lost.

No matter what time of day you choose to run, be sure to do some of your training, particularly your longer runs, at the same time of day as you will be running your marathon. You want those runs to simulate marathon training as much as possible, and your body does get used to performing at a specific time of day. (For proof, just try exercising at a time you are unaccustomed to, and see how difficult it can be.)

While there is a great advantage to being flexible, we are creatures of habit, and the body does seem to have an internal clock. You will likely find comfort and a sense of discipline in a predictable training routine. Jumbo Elliott, the legendary Villanova University track coach, used to tell his many champion runners, "Live like a clock." Run the same, eat the same, and sleep the same.

For at least half my career, I worked full time as a schoolteacher (with a two-hour commute) and ran full time as well. People thought I was crazy. Now there is so much more understanding of and respect for running, so you will likely get a lot of support from people when they know you are training for a marathon. Back in my day, I found it hard to ask people for support, but you do need moral support, especially when you are training for a marathon. You're making a big commitment, and while the world (and the people in it you live and work with) can't come to a halt for you, it's reasonable to request some help or flexibility.

WHAT TO DO IF YOU'RE ON THE ROAD

Chances are good that in the course of your preparation, you may find yourself outside your normal training environment. Whether a business meeting or trip, or a family vacation, there will likely be times you'll be challenged to stick to the program. But while you may be on vacation, you shouldn't take a vacation from running. If you do, you need to have planned ahead to build more weeks into your program. Get right back on track when you return home.

To stick to your schedule when you are in a foreign place, however, can take a lot of discipline. If your job requires travel, you'll be tested. Try to engage your coworkers in a run, even if the primary purpose is to explore the city. Chances are you will gain their respect just for asking. If you don't feel comfortable braving new surroundings and don't mind a treadmill, check out the hotel gym. Also, if you can, plan your trip either very early (when the necessary mileage is lower) or much later in your race preparation. When you are more fully committed, you may be more motivated and disciplined to stay with your routine.

I met John Stanton several years ago on a visit to the Ottawa Marathon in 2004. I was very impressed with his running store and his training groups, one of which I attended. I was in awe of how organized and inspiring he was. A remarkable number of people showed up for the training group, and they were really relying on John to help them get through the marathon.

JOHN STANTON: Since I founded the Running Room in Canada twenty-one years ago, I have had over 600,000 people go through our walking and running programs. Every time I'm out with a group, about 90 percent of those preparing for a marathon are first-timers. All you have to do is look at the burgeoning growth of the event to understand it. It not only changes them, it empowers them. There is something very special in seeing that. You see the personal strength, the confidence, as their body posture improves. You get their sense of purpose. That's what training for a marathon does. In my experience, for every marathoner that finishes, it's not so much the medal and the celebration. It's even bigger. It's that if you have an intelligent goal, and a group of supporters, you can do anything in life.

MEETING THE CHALLENGE

Many people read about getting fit, running, and doing a marathon. But the true test is in the action, the ability to say, "Yes, I can do this." The resources to help you run are plentiful, but the inner will has to come from within. Often I hear, I'm too old, too tall, too thin, or too fat. But people of every ability, or disability, have various reasons that get them started running—from weight control to smoking cessation to overcoming a disaster, like divorce or the loss of a loved one. These are all good reasons to take control of your life. That's what you do when you decide to run a marathon.

The marathon has been referred to as a person's horizontal Everest. It answers the question: What's the next challenge? It's kind of the ultimate, going beyond the ordinary. Goal-setting and self-satisfaction are important. But what's even more critical is that the marathon builds a sense of community in a time when our world really needs it. When we toe the line, we are all there as athletes. Whether you're the Kenyan trying to break 2:06 or you finish in six hours, we respect one another: the six-hour person for the speed of the Kenyan, and the Kenyan for the tenacity of the six-hour person. At the same time, we're participating in a sport both of us love.

But it isn't necessarily easy to reach the marathon goal. Visualization is very important in this quest. Often when we start an exercise program or decide to do a marathon, we ask ourselves: "How did I get into this?" Particularly if you start to feel fatigue during the race, you question yourself. That's why I recommend some power words. It helps a lot to create a mantra, something like, "I'm strong. I'm fit. I've trained hard for this. I believe in myself. I know I can do this." This deflects physical discomfort, moves you beyond it, and allows you to stay positive. If you can talk your way through it, you'll start to feel better.

The way I see the marathon, you are an actor who is going through yet another rehearsal (like your training runs), but this time with a crowd to cheer you on. Everything you do on race day should have been rehearsed in training: learning to run tired, take in food and fluids, run hills, run in a group—it's all been practiced. That way, the race isn't a test; it's a celebration. The test has already been passed—on the hot, humid days or the cold days you've trained through. The race is graduation day. You're going to get your medal, get your picture taken. So take it all in.

BURNOUT

In all the excitement of planning a marathon, people can't imagine getting burned out. But it happens.

To their credit, some people are very dedicated and disciplined. But that can also mean they are rigid, and rigidity puts them at risk. I had days when

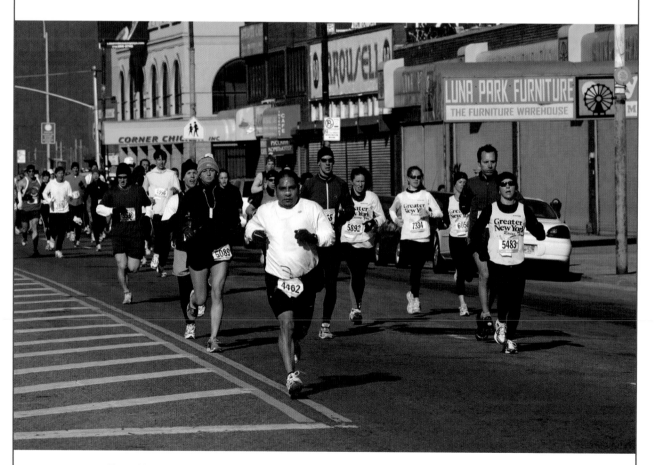

Everything you do during your training, including your lifestyle choices, prepares you for the big day.

I was pressured or exhausted, when running meant going out in the cold and dark before commuting to work, or when my husband Jack would force me to skip a session. That was very tough for me, since I live by routine. Using my diary did help, though. I was able to gain a sense of security that I had done enough and that taking off the occasional session when I needed to was the right thing to do.

Looking back, I should have been even more flexible. That's why I tell people that if they have a long run planned and they're overly tired, wait until they feel more rested. I should have listened to my body more than my guilt. If you need to take off, do it. Don't risk burning out. If you've planned ahead, you can afford a break. If burnout does strike, take an easy week or two to recover your energy and enthusiasm. Then, start up your program where you left off.

Most of you have jobs, responsibilities, and busy lives. Marathon training is not your full-time occupation. It has to share time. In my line of work, I meet all kinds of people and all kinds of runners. Some are overstressed and obsessed. Others are like my brother Jan, who takes everything in stride. He knows what he has to do and gets the training done. Gimmicks, like miracle training programs or fad diets, don't distract him. He even likes a good party before the marathon. But he still manages to do one of them a year and has done so successfully for the past twenty years.

Don't be a slave to the program. I can't stress this enough when I speak to groups. You have your own personal rhythms, and you also have to factor in what's going on in your life. Too many people separate their training from their work or family. Training is comprised of various components: nutrition, training, rest, and recovery. If you cheat on one of these parts, you compromise achieving your end goal.

Boredom and staleness aren't exactly burnout, but do contribute to it. Everyone needs some variety once in a while. If you feel stale, perhaps as a result of doing too much of the same thing, try mixing it up a little. Run some different courses, with difference scenery and new people, or, if you feel you can, mix up the times of day when you run. Sometimes even a simple change in routine can be refreshing.

ARE YOU OVERTRAINING?

One prominent cause of burnout is overtraining. In my experience, most people associate overtraining with serious, or world class, athletes. After all, you may reason, how can you overtrain if you are being provided with an authoritative, sensible training program, one which also allows the flexibility to take days off? However, even the most reasonable training program can create problems if it is more than your body or lifestyle can handle.

You need to be on the lookout for signs of overtraining. In addition to obvious symptoms like fatigue, tired legs, or illness, there are other signs, such as: persistent muscle soreness that doesn't go away even after you are warmed

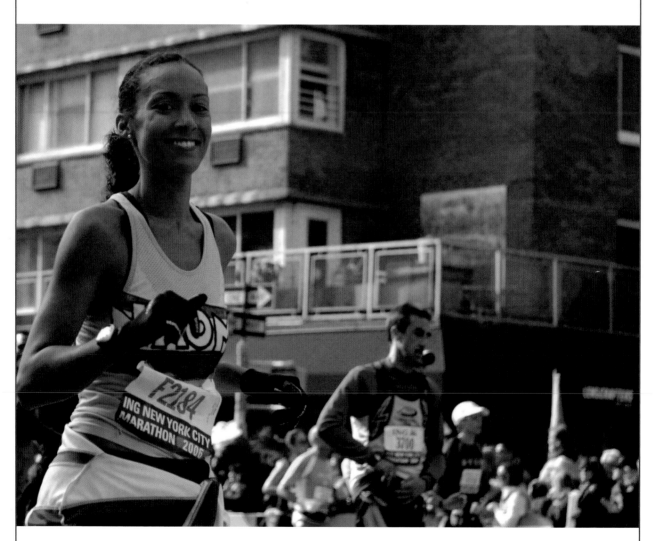

You should feel fresh and enthusiastic to run. Beware of the "blahs," potentially a sign of overtraining.

up, uncharacteristic moodiness, short temper or irritability; insomnia or loss of appetite; or a morning heart rate elevated by five to ten beats.

If you have any of these symptoms, it is safest to cut back and recover. Ignoring or pushing through them carries all kinds of risks. Overtraining increases the likelihood of illness or injury. The body is a wonderful machine when it comes to taking care of itself; if you push it too far, it will eventually shut down. On the other hand, if you rest when you should, it will recover and get stronger.

To get through 26.2 miles, you've got to be up for the preparation. Training stops being satisfying when you are stale. Try to avoid the trap of overtraining in the first place by careful planning (such as proper spacing of your days off from running) and by monitoring your body's response to training. (Use your training diary to assist you.) If you have overtrained or are faced with the challenge of injury, take the necessary steps to deal with it.

If you do fall victim to overtraining, don't punish yourself. Accept that it is a learning experience, and vow to make your recovery quick and complete. Think positively about resting: it is good for you and is the best road to recovery. (Trust me; you will soon forget the days you have to take off, if you make sure to take them early, at the onset of a problem, so time off is minimal.) Use your recovery time to pamper yourself (warm baths, good nutrition, extra sleep). This will recharge you mentally as well as physically, so you will be optimally ready to go again. Finally, make sure to start back conservatively. Don't begin with one of your long runs. Test yourself first with some of the shorter runs. Make up whatever time you missed by going back to the week where you left off, if you have scheduled a few extra buffer weeks before the marathon.

9

Mental Motivators

Frank Horwill advises the members of the Serpentine Running Club, comprised of about 2,500 runners of all abilities in central London. In an article on the club's Web site, the coach states that the difference between a good club runner and an Olympic champion is not really that great. "It is in their mental attitude that the difference occurs," he concludes. Imagine that mental potential—one which we all have—acting for you. Among the qualities that Horwill claims stand out in his Olympians are ones that you can embody as well. His champions never missed a training session. As their training got harder, their belief in regards to performance increased. They had a sense of humor. And they kept at it: a bad result was not a catastrophe, but a reason to be more determined.

As the noted saying goes—training is 90 percent physical and 10 percent mental, but look out for that 10 percent. You are about to undertake something you've never done, to enter territory you've never inhabited. You will soon discover how important "mind power" is to your new endeavor.

What spurs the kind of positive motivation that Frank Horwill finds in his champions? This is a key question that can unlock an important door for you. Making the initial decision to run a marathon is the easy part. It's the follow-up that proves to be a challenge. Previously, I mentioned my nephew, Terje, my brother Jan's son. When he vowed to run a marathon in late 2007, I had trouble believing him because he was overweight and not in running shape. "I'm going to do it," he told me. "I'm really motivated." I waited for the winter snow to melt, to see if he began more serious training than chasing after his son's soccer ball. I was surprised to see he was well on his way. Although I joke it's the bet he's made with his father that motivates him, I think most people benefit more from internal drive.

Many people assume they can do more than they can. They want the glory without the hard work. I meet would-be marathoners, who tell me, "I thought I was in better shape. I didn't think it would be so hard." They do little to prepare and yet feel they are in great shape. But give them a more structured program that demands more effort, and they fold. It's not always so easy to devote oneself to marathon training. There are all kinds of reasons we can all find that make it too difficult.

But these mental barriers are by no means insurmountable. "Mental motivators" will not only help you to overcome barriers both in training and during the race, they may help you avoid them in the first place. And as you obviously realize, they are valuable skills to use in many other endeavors in life.

VISUALIZATION

Visualization, also called positive imagery, means mentally picturing yourself achieving your goals. Visualization reinforces a positive attitude and helps you to focus. It also helps you to achieve a desired outcome. Visualization is more than just a "mind game"; it can actually improve your performance. Many studies prove this. Athletes in various sports have been tested at rest, visualizing their performances. Their muscles actually created the physical response to their sport activity.

To give it a try, start by paying attention to your form—your dropped and relaxed shoulders, your arm swing, your stride. Feel your feet hitting the pavement and your even breathing. Feel the wind hitting your face, blowing through your hair. The more specific and detailed your visualization, the better it works. You can also use visualization when you rest, like a meditation. As a first-time marathoner, you should spend time visualizing yourself getting ready, being on the starting line, and seeing yourself finishing, feeling good. Put your focus on the positive aspects associated with the race. You may not naturally visualize in such detail early in your training or for your shorter training runs, but as the race gets closer, you will automatically begin to visualize, like daydreaming. I always visualized in order to give me motivation during my hard workouts. I would see myself around other runners and imagine myself on the specific race course.

If for any reason negative thoughts creep into your visualization (such as fatigue, apprehension, or a poor outcome), don't be distressed. It's good practice and an important part of the training process to learn to force the negativity away by replacing it with more positive thoughts. My career wasn't all success. I certainly had my challenges—times of self-doubt when I visualized poor outcomes. If I didn't do well in a race, it was publicized in big newspaper headlines, for all to see. I admit that affected my confidence. When times got tough, I used visualization to focus on my intense desire to redeem myself and do well in my next race. If you do visualize adversity, don't attempt to push it away. Rather, picture yourself overcoming any obstacle.

FOCUS

During my running days, I concentrated so deeply that I was often completely unaware of my surroundings. In fact, my training partners—my brothers or Jack—had to be there to warn me, or I'd run right through puddles or potholes. I learned this intense concentration by running on the track, where the race goes by so quickly, you can't afford to lose focus for even a second. Also, even in training, the track oval, with its precision measurements and lack of distraction, lends itself to forcing you to focus.

You're likely to spend a good portion of your training, and perhaps your race, chatting with others, or letting your mind wander—and that's fine. It should be an enjoyable experience. But part of the experience is also learning to concentrate and to focus on your running when necessary. This focus is particularly important in the latter stage of a long run, or during the actual marathon. It is also important for you to focus in order to monitor your effort and your body.

Your focus may also vary depending on the circumstances in your daily life. You may find that training is an ideal time to sort out your schedule, or think about your problems. Similar to visualization, it's difficult to focus on the marathon in your first week of training, when running 26.2 miles seems an alien concept. However, focus will become more automatic when you are out on the roads for a few hours and also when you practice by running a race or two at an intermediate distance.

Just as sometimes running is physically different, it should sometimes be mentally different. Focus on what is appropriate to each session. As Horwill points out, "The adrenal system secretes hormones for physical activity to be undertaken." Some sessions are stressful, and some are for recovery. "Press the right key in your brain to bring about the appropriate physical reaction. If it's going to be tough, tell yourself so. "This is going to be tough. I need a resolute

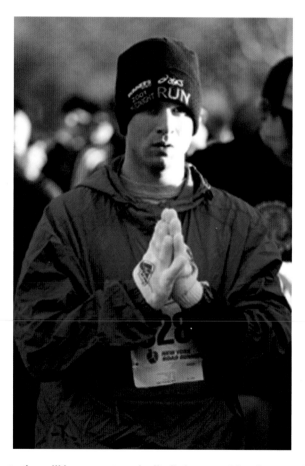

Intense concentration will happen automatically. Embrace and develop your ability to focus on your effort.

attitude." Or, "This is a recovery run. I can afford to look around at the trees or people in the park."

SELF-CONFIDENCE

Although training prepares you physically, a trained mind (including an understanding of what your body may be going through) is what gives you the self-confidence to get you through the race. While you may be able to fake confidence in other endeavors in life, you can't fool yourself in the marathon. You have to build the attitude, "I can do it." If you are programmed to believe in your success, you will achieve it. It has been proven time and again that we are what we think, and we achieve what we believe we are capable of achieving.

NO PAIN, NO GAIN

People don't like to bring up the subject of pain, especially with beginners, because they think it will discourage them, or that it is associated with a type of running they should not be doing. I have a different way of looking at physical effort. It's "positive pain." I think you will be much better prepared for the challenge of the race if you learn to accept the effort (as opposed to calling it pain) and overcome your fear of discomfort. When you realize you can be in control of your effort, of the fatigue or pain, it becomes a "friendly" pain. If you do get to the point where the discomfort feels overwhelming, and if you have practiced your mental skills, your mind will help you in ways even your body can't. Also, it helps to understand you are not alone. If you look at your running partner or group, or glance around in the race—especially in the later miles—you'll realize that everyone is working hard, pushing through the pain. This is part of the experience and part of the camaraderie. If you watch people finishing races, you'll see plenty of pain. But you'll also notice that it's usually the tired runners, bent over in fatigue, who are the ones reaching out to shake hands or embrace each other in congratulations.

There are several other motivators that, while not necessarily springing from your mind, nevertheless assist your motivation from a psychological point of view.

MAKING USE OF FRIENDS AND GROUPS

As John Stanton points out, "The days of the solitary long distance runner in the 1970s and '80s are over." Although I did my share of running alone, I am fortunate I grew up in a culture with sports clubs, where we mostly trained in a group. (I have belonged to a club called Vidar since I was a child.) Also, I come from a running family, so I have always had my husband or my brothers to help get me out the door and on the run.

Partners or groups provide camaraderie, fun, and positive peer pressure. When you train with like-minded individuals, and perhaps make new friends, that helps keep you going. Running partners become sensitive to each other's needs, chatting and pulling each other along when necessary. While you can likely manage on your own for the shorter training runs, it is most helpful to be accompanied by friends on your long runs. If you don't have a running partner or a group, try to come up with creative support, such as having your children ride bicycles while you run or finding someone to meet you along the way to give you water, nourishment, and some words of encouragement.

RUN FOR A CAUSE

You are embarking on a satisfying mission, despite its inevitable challenges along the way. There is another way to keep your motivation, and your

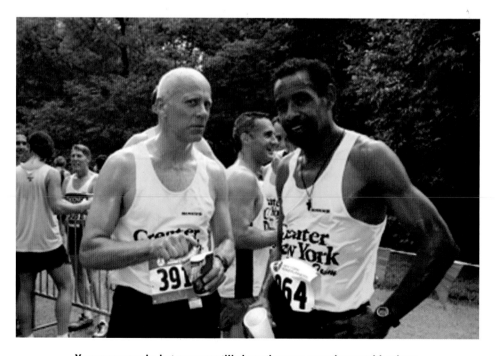

You may run solo, but you can still share the race experience with others.

inspiration, strong. Stanton endorses at least fifty charities on his Running Room Web site. He says that one of the most fundamental reasons charity running is so popular is because it gives us positive reinforcement for running—beyond just ourselves. "When we are training for a marathon, and even in the midst of the race, we all go through periods of self-doubt, but having a cause will allow you to dig deep within yourself, and to make it to the finish line," he says. Stanton, who advises that you choose a charity close to yourself or your beliefs, also feels that bonding to a cause serves an even larger purpose. "At times like these, when our world can seem in disarray, running for charity helps build a sense of community and purpose."

I've always been impressed by the commitment of those who run for a charity, which I first experienced in the London Marathon in the 1980s. Also, many charities have group training. You belong to their organization, and you get a lot of support, in terms both of training advice and being together with others who share a common goal. Since 1995, I've been team captain for Fred's Team (named for the late race director, Fred Lebow), which raises money for cancer research. When I got sick with cancer myself, they dedicated their 2005 New York City Marathon to me and raised over two million dollars. I was honored and touched.

> *Michael Franfurt has been my attorney and financial guide since my early days of marathoning. He's always been "laid back" but serious about running and competing in his age group. He's in good shape and still keeps up an impressive running and racing schedule. He's an inspiration for us all as we get older.*
>
> MIKE FRANFURT: If I were to come up with a first-time marathon headline, it would be "I'll never do it again, or, now I know I can do anything." That was what the experience was like for me. My first marathon was coincidentally on Earth Day, March, 1974. After a nineteen-year layoff from running since college, I was moving my body again as a forty-year-old. I had done some road races, and after three months of inadequate training, and having run an eighteen- and a twenty-miler, I figured, "Okay, I can run a marathon." And off I went. It was a hot, muggy day on Long Island. I was making my way around lovely Eisenhower Park, thinking, "This is pretty easy." But by the fourth time around, with four miles to go, I went into slow motion. There was no more water on the course, and I was dehydrated. I clearly remember a beautiful woman passing me. It was the famed women's distance running pioneer, Nina

Kuscsik. I asked her, "How much further to go?" She answered four miles, but I mumbled and swore it was only two. I didn't realize that I was hallucinating from the dehydration. We came past a bathroom in the middle of the park. "There's water in there," I thought. But the door was locked. I asked one of the other runners to boost me onto the roof, to get in and get some water. He just kept on running.

Somehow, I made it to the last turn of the track. At that point, what felt like two bullets entered into my hamstrings, and my legs spasmed. I simply couldn't go forward. So, walking backwards, I very dutifully crossed the finish line. I felt like one of Washington's troops at Valley Forge. I was in total distress, almost a corpse. Someone said to me, "You only missed qualifying for Boston by thirty-one seconds, but if you write a letter, they'll let you in." "You gotta be crazy," I shot back, "I'll never do this thing again in my life!" A half hour later, I was in my motel. My legs still weren't working, so I went up the stairs backwards, on my rear end. I had a few beers, and by then, it suddenly flashed through my mind: "I can do anything. I just ran a marathon." And I started talking about doing another one.

After that first marathon, I went on to do forty-nine more. On the day of my sixtyth birthday, I did my fiftyth, and last. I crossed the finish line and announced to my beautiful wife that I was retired from marathoning. That was eleven years ago. I continue to run and enjoy shorter races, but my memories of my first marathon are still vivid.

So, when you cross that finish line, the revelation you have is my sage advice: What more is there in life than a moment when you know you can do anything?

10

Shoes and More

Outside of training, shopping for shoes is undoubtedly the most important preparation you will make for your marathon.

"My favorite customers are first-time marathoners, because they have no preconceived ideas," says John Fabbro, owner of Fleet Feet Sports, a running store and mecca in Montclair, New Jersey. Fabbro, himself an experienced marathoner, has personally assisted thousands of those new to the event during the twenty years he has owned and operated the store.

Fabbro makes this claim because runners are compelled to adapt to changing times. Footwear is constantly evolving, to the benefit of those who are savvy consumers. It is not uncommon that a model you enjoy may be revamped in a mere six months. And if the new version does not suit you well, you may discover an entirely new model.

It pays to go to a running specialty store, especially if you are relatively new to running. That's because a good salesperson shouldn't just ask you your size and then bring out a bunch of pairs of shoes. Fabbro operates by the Fleet Feet "fitlosophy," a system of serving customers that includes a dialogue to determine key factors in shoe selection, such as goals, running surfaces, and what he or she likes or dislikes about past shoes. In fact, he claims that one out of four customers say they have had some sort of shoe trouble or concern.

In my experience, when it comes to shoes, don't depend on what others have to say. They may recommend a great shoe, but what works for one person may not be right for you. Running shoes depend greatly on individual taste. A lot of runners in clinics ask for my shoe recommendations. I always tell them the best approach is to find a good salesperson to help them.

Shoes should be inconspicuous. That's the bottom line according to Fabbro: "Our goal is to make footwear a non-issue—that the shoe is so comfortable that you don't even think about it, until it's worn out and needs to be replaced." He has some suggestions for what to look for when shoe shopping.

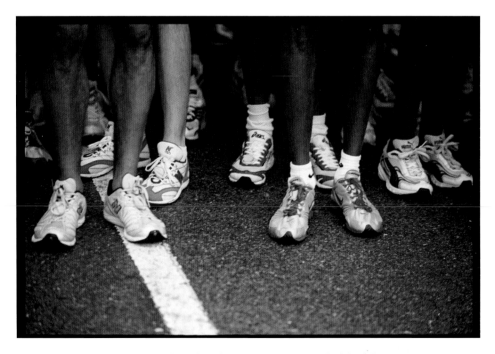

Make sure to break in your shoes in training before the race. And don't forget to "test run" your race socks and clothing as well.

Bring in Your Old Shoes

This includes those you've run or even walked in. These shoes serve as a "road map," providing footwear patterns that are important clues for the salesperson. The same holds true for the socks you wear.

Try on Shoes with Running Socks

Socks make a big difference. A very thick sock, for example, can add as much as a half size to your shoe.

Have Your Feet Properly Measured

Fabbro uses the classic metal foot measurer you may recognize from your childhood. It's called a Brannock Device. Instead of measuring the foot only one way, Fabbro believes it is best to measure the foot first without bearing weight and then again while bearing weight to determine how the arch functions when the foot is planted. This analysis determines the size, width, and style of the shoe best suited to you. It also determines what degree of support you will need, depending on how stable (rigid) or collapsible your arch is. Optionally, or together with the use of the Brannock Device, an experienced salesperson may examine your feet (or even touch them), or watch how you walk or run. Some even have treadmills in the store for this purpose. The salesperson may take you outside to observe your foot plant while you run to evaluate how the shoe supports your foot.

Choose a Shoe That Supports, Not Distorts, the Foot

The shoes you choose should feel fairly natural during heel-to-toe movement; i.e., moving through your stride, without lumps, bumps, or other distractions or abnormalities.

Try on at Least Two to Three Pairs of Shoes for Contrast

You don't need the dealer to bring out the whole back room (a dozen pairs is overkill), but even if the first pair of shoes out of the box feels perfect, you should try on some other pairs for comparison. Put one shoe from each pair on for the best contrast.

Buy Your Shoes Big Enough

Fabbro says that probably the biggest mistake those shopping without professional advice make is to buy shoes that are too small. Your feet will expand during long-distance runs. A properly fitted shoe allows a half to one thumb width of space from the end of your longest toe (not necessarily your big toe). There is no standard in manufacturers' sizes, so don't go by the number—choose by the fit.

Consider Investing in Two Pairs of Shoes

Ideally, Fabbro wants his customers to run in a new pair of shoes, analyze the experience, and then invest in a second pair—especially before the first pair wears out. He suggests purchasing a different model for the second pair, but with similar features to the shoes you like. This allows one pair to completely dry out after use. And because the shoes offer a different fit, the second pair somewhat alters the stress on the foot, therefore changing the stress on the entire body.

Plan to Spend Between $85 and $100

"Just because the shoe is more expensive doesn't mean it's better for you. It all comes down to fit," says Fabbro, who also warns against being too frugal. His store doesn't carry shoes under $80.

Check Out Insoles

A wide variety of over-the-counter insoles are top sellers these days, says Fabbro. You might consider checking them out if your foot elongates more than one full shoe size when planted. Insoles were originally marketed to help prevent typical runners' injuries, such as plantar fasciitis (strain on the ligament in the foot). You can always start with the insole that comes with the shoe and, if necessary, replace it with one of the sturdier over-the-counter models later.

Pay Attention to the Lifespan of the Shoe

Shoes last from between 350 to 500 miles, but as the marathon draws closer, if you can afford it, Fabbro advises you to get a new pair for the race. Make sure to break them in by running in them for at least a part of your training the month before the event.

SHOE CATEGORIES

The basic categories of shoes from which to choose are:

Lightweight Trainer

You should probably shy away from this style as a first-time marathoner. It doesn't offer enough support.

Neutral Cushioning

This is meant for a high-arched and somewhat rigid foot (i.e., a foot that does not excessively elongate when you step down).

Stability

Eighty percent of Fabbro's customers buy this category of shoe. "It's the sedan of shoes," he says, "the most value for your money."

Motion Control

This is a more heavy-duty shoe, for those with a significant amount of foot elongation and pronation (i.e., feet tilt inwards when running or walking).

SOCKS

Wearing a great shoe with a cheap sock does a disservice to the shoe, claims Fabbro. A cheap sock is made of coarser materials, which can cause "hot spots," eventually leading to blisters. A good sock fits snuggly against your skin, hugging the foot, without gaps. Thick or thin, long or short—it's fine to go with personal preference. However, invest in a good quality sock, which should cost $7 to $12 and can last up to eighteen months. In evaluating the quality of the sock, the thickness of the yarn is less important than a high needle count. You can tell that by looking on the inside of the sock. The more loops and the closer together they are, the higher the needle count, and the less the sock will compress over time. Even good running socks, in my experience, can still cause problems. If anything on the inside of the sock bothers me, I run with them turned inside out, even if I have to stop mid-run in order to reverse them.

CLOTHING

Despite the warnings about cotton—that once you sweat, you're wet—Fabbro claims even the most experienced runners can still be seen wearing old T-shirts for running (souvenirs from races, for example). That might do for short runs in temperate weather, but for the long haul, and for the marathon itself, you'll want performance wear. This gear is mostly made of polyester fibers that are meant to keep you warm in the cold and cool in the heat, by wicking away moisture from the skin. This clothing also keeps you dry. "You lose heat from the body twenty times faster when you're wet than when you're dry," says Fabbro. This fabric can be found in head-to-toe gear, from shorts and shirts to visors, hats, and socks. If you're planning on carrying nutritional gels or other necessities when you run, check out running shorts that are made with special pockets for storage purposes.

If you run in darkness, or even near darkness, invest in extra reflective gear. Even though small amounts of reflective strips come on shoes or shorts, to be properly visible, a special lightweight reflective vest or blinking light is a must.

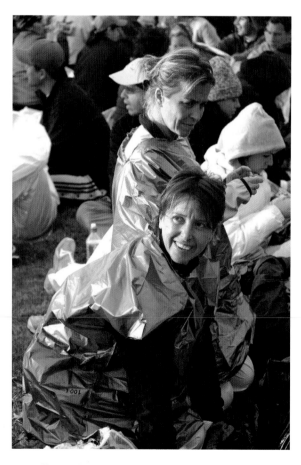

Prepare to keep yourself warm however you can. Plastic garbage bags, discarded before the race, are customary items worn while waiting at the marathon start.

SPORTS BRAS

The days of "the one size fits all, pull over your head" running bras are long gone. If you're bigger than a B cup, you shouldn't choose the shapeless model. Excessive bouncing is not only uncomfortable; it can stretch ligaments, which do not return to their original shape. If you are larger, go for a more supportive bra, one that encapsulates the breasts. Like conventional bras, these bras hook in the back and may also feature adjustable Velcro straps. Women tend to hold onto their sports bras past their material's prime. (The bra's elastic wears out.) The rule of thumb for bra wear is to buy a new bra each time you purchase new running shoes, and throw out your oldest one. Obviously, bras should not constrict, or rub the skin. Test them by trying them on before buying and running in place in the dressing room. Run your fingers over any seams or lumps to make sure they won't chafe.

GADGETS

If you're considering buying a heart rate monitor (HRM), shop around. Speak to experts in running or sports stores. Some HRMs are very fancy and measure and analyze every aspect of training; these require the use of a computer to calculate the data. This is probably overkill. Such devices usually advertise that they are for the serious or elite athlete. A basic device (which can still include some extra features, such as a calorie counter) shouldn't cost more than $100.

Some people use a car odometer to measure a running route; then there's Googleearth.com (see explanation in Chapter 6). If you want to be able to accurately monitor your pace as well as the distance you have covered while you are running, however, you will need a GPS device. This gadget can cost about $250. Personally, I don't feel one of these is necessary. Beyond a certain point, technology can become excessive. As I've mentioned, training is not an exact science, nor should determining your pace or distance have to be. Also, there is the important element of getting to know your own body and negotiating your training accordingly.

There are various other useful items you can check out. "On long runs, you start to notice things like chafing," points out John Fabbro. Nipple guards (NipGuards) for men prevent chafing (you can also use Band-Aids). Chafing can also be solved by an inexpensive anti-chafing lubricant marketed to athletes, also used for feet or underarms, which is a big seller. Petroleum jelly will also solve this problem. Although I made do without carrying drink bottles for most of my career (although I did eventually try a belt with small water bottles), newer models of drink-on-the-run equipment are now available. Some feature a small bag worn on the waist (called a bladder pack), with

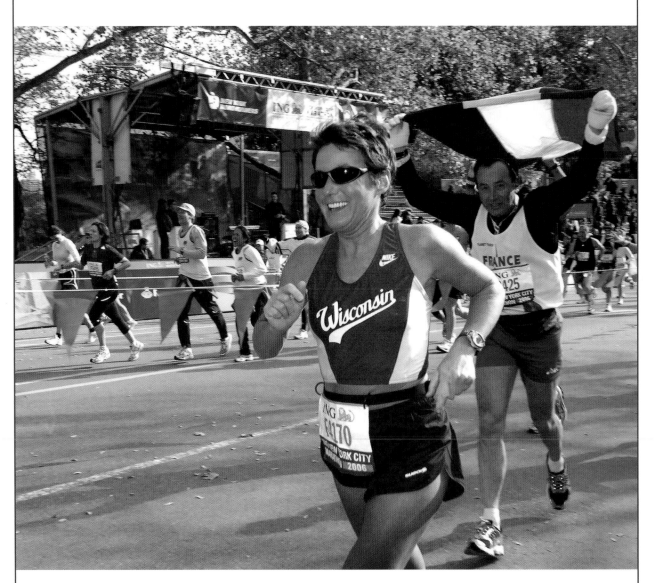

Protect your eyes with lightweight sports sunglasses. (Don't forget to apply sunscreen as well. The sun gets through even on cloudy days.)

the bag carried on the lower back, featuring a tube to drink from, similar to a straw. Some of these packs also offer storage space for gels and bars.

Shoe and gear shopping should not be overly complicated or very expensive, especially when compared to the cost of other activities. John Fabbro's philosophy is to keep things simple. "Add layers of confusion only as you need them," he concludes.

11
Staying Healthy

For over twenty years, I was relatively injury-free, until the last three years of my career, when I got a couple of stress fractures. Even these could have been avoided if I had stopped running earlier, at the onset of the warning signs (beginning with soreness). But I was a "runner," and in those days, that meant as long as you can run, you do. That is, until the warnings become so severe, you have no choice but to stop. I wasn't smart; I didn't learn. So now I tell people what I found out the hard way, so that they can learn from my example.

In the late 1990s, I met David Lowenthal, M.D., Ph.D., in Gainesville, Florida, where we were both runners seeking care from our mutual friend, noted Irish sports physical therapist Gerard Hartmann. Dr. Lowenthal has wide professional and personal experience in the area of running, health, and fitness. He is a professor of medicine pharmacology and exercise science at the

University of Florida College of Medicine and College of Health and Human Performance in Gainesville, and Director Emeritus, Geriatric Research, Education and Clinical Center at the Department of Veteran's Administration, also in Gainesville. Notably, he has also completed fifteen marathons, with a best time of 3:40.

Medical care goes hand in hand with your marathon program. In that vein, it should be first steps first, says Dr. Lowenthal. Anyone who has been sedentary should consult with a physician before undertaking an exercise program. He is also most adamant that beginning marathoners or exercisers, no matter what age, should use this opportunity to identify their health profile, specifically any covert or overt cardiovascular risk factors they might have, either personally or genetically. This means such markers as elevated blood pressure, cardiac arrhythmias, blood sugar, fasting blood sugar (a 2-hour blood sugar) and a hemoglobin A1C, and lipids (HDL and LDL: that is, levels of good and bad cholesterol). Exercise, such as running, can help lower blood pressure and abnormal lipids (bad cholesterol), but often it does not take care of these problems in a timely manner and can exacerbate other health problems.

"This workup gets into preventive medicine, which is a critical point," says Dr. Lowenthal, who directs prospective runners to make an appointment with an M.D. internist to hone in on any potential risk factors. Also, he advises that you tell the doctor about any medications you are taking; some, such as beta-blockers or diuretics, could interfere with the normal responses to exercise. Diuretics may cause disturbances in blood electrolytes. A beta-blocker slows the heart rate, so judging a runner's heart rate response can be quite difficult.

PREVENTION IS KEY

While there are methods of pain relief as well as medical diagnosis and help, what should be emphasized, in Dr. Lowenthal's opinion (and my opinion as well), is preventive measures against injury, such as stretching to ensure flexibility; strength training to balance any muscular weaknesses; and cross training, such as stationary biking, to relieve the impact the feet, knees, and hips incur during running. This applies especially to those with pain in those areas and stiffness upon awakening, most often in people over 50. Also, follow a sensible and methodical approach to training, as is laid out in the guidelines and training programs in the book, to help you avoid injury.

WHAT TO DO IF YOU ARE IN PAIN

"The old dogma of 'no pain, no gain' is something I do not subscribe to," says Dr. Lowenthal. "Pain is your body telling you that you've done too much, and/or something is injured. If you sustain an injury, the first symptom you might perceive is pain. This should be a red flag warning to stop what you are doing. If the pain is new and different than you've had before, it is prudent to see a physician who deals in sports medicine." However, you shouldn't wait if it is head, chest, or abdominal pain. The sudden onset of chest pain should be immediately evaluated in an ER and not ignored or ascribed to training.

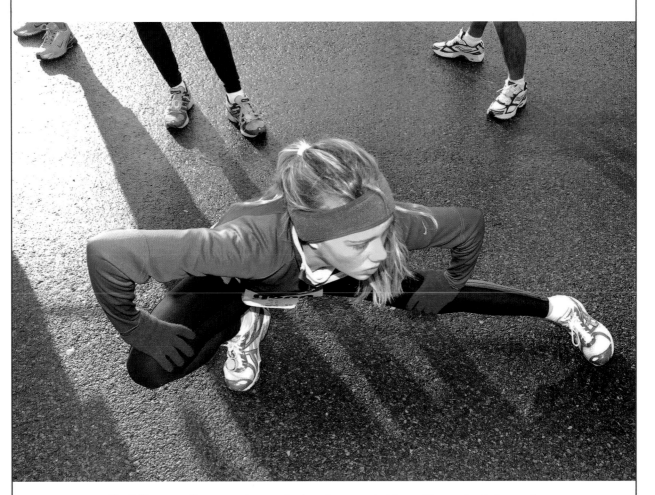

Flexibility, as well as general strengthening of areas not addressed by running, helps you to achieve the necessary balanced fitness.

You will likely have to rest for as long as the pain takes to go away, says Dr. Lowenthal, who adds that you can use ice or over-the-counter medications (such as ibuprofen) for pain relief. But when you use these measures, he recommends also making an appointment with a doctor.

Beware that the use of over-the-counter pain medication can also impact other aspects of your health, so it is best to understand your health profile, first with an exam that tests cardiovascular risk factors. Also, Dr. Lowenthal points out, this medication can mask the true problem, often related to overtraining. In some instances, NSAIDS (Non-Steroidal Anti-Inflammatory Drugs; e.g., ibuprofen or Naprosyn) can increase blood pressure and decrease kidney function, and mask serious injuries like stress fractures.

Also, the older you are when you begin exercising, the greater the risk for soft tissue or bone and joint injuries. This is why it is important to get in shape very gradually and thoroughly before undertaking a marathon program. And marathon training, in and of itself, does carry risks; the more training mileage, the greater the chance of injury.

TYPICAL RUNNING INJURIES

"Runners are an intelligent group of people. They often believe that if they are injured, they can make a diagnosis and then treat it," says Dr. Lowenthal, who cautions against any such self-diagnosis. However, that does not mean that the various lower body injuries typical to runners should not be well understood. The information below is a very basic sample; the purpose is not to cover every injury, but to highlight some of the typical potential problem areas.

Most major marathons have extensive medical teams stationed at the start, along the course, and at the finish. Also, medical personnel are often available for consultation at the race Expo. Make sure to take advantage of them if you have any concerns or problems.

FEET

Dr. Lowenthal points out that one classic runner's problem can be felt immediately upon awakening in the morning and when standing barefoot. It is a pain in the sole of the foot, called plantar fasciitis, which is an inflammation of the soft tissue that usually begins with the sole of the foot and heel and advances to the Achilles tendon and travels over the heel—like a fan spreading out. It is caused by overuse. "A good podiatrist will suggest an over-the-counter shoe insert for support, which can be worn for forty-five to sixty minutes at a time," says Dr. Lowenthal, who cautions against immediate investment in costly custom-made orthotics. He also suggests ice therapy and seeing a physical therapist for some deep tissue massage.

Dr. Lowenthal speaks from personal experience. After a recent bout of plantar fasciitis, he was treated by a physical therapist and instructed to do only non-weight bearing workouts. He used a stationary bike, and his foot took about eight weeks to heal. He was especially strict with his rehabilitation, since he says this injury is associated with a strong degree of recurrence.

Another related injury is Achilles tendinitis (inflammation of the Achilles tendon). One indication of this condition is that the pain occurs when the foot is flexed upwards (toward the nose). Medical confirmation is necessary, however, to determine that it is Achilles tendinitis. This is one of the injuries that can be prevented with adequate stretching and strengthening. Standing on a step and letting your heel drop until you feel a stretch in the calves is one method. This stretch can also help prevent plantar fasciitis. (See the exercise for Heel Drops in Chapter 7).

BLISTERS

A seemingly small glitch such as a blister can become debilitating, especially if it occurs during a marathon. The key to blisters is to prevent them in the first place, by making sure your feet stay dry, wearing properly fitted shoes and socks, and taking care to protect toes or bony protrusions on your feet with padding. If you feel a "hot spot," or irritation, the use of an anti-chafing product should help. However, if after using these measures a blister does develop, drain it with a sterile pin, leave the skin on, apply an antibiotic ointment, and cover the blister with one of the over-the-counter products used for blister protection. These products are also useful if you experience the beginnings of a blister. When Gloria ran the New York City Marathon, she took advantage of one of the many helpful features of the race—volunteers held out wooden sticks coated with petroleum jelly. Worried that a "hot spot" indicated a blister was developing, she stopped briefly at mile fifteen, took off her shoes and socks, and applied the jelly. She finished the race blister-free.

The longer you've been running, and the more miles you run, the greater the risk is for a foot injury. Sufficient pounding can result in a non-life threatening hemorrhage underneath the toenail, called a subungual hematoma, or accumulation of blood. This is so painful that you will need a podiatrist, or even an ER visit, to treat it. "After the 1979 Boston Marathon, I could barely walk back to my hotel," relates Dr. Lowenthal. A podiatrist poked a hole in his toenail to alleviate the pressure, after which he experienced immediate relief. This condition differs from black toenail (or "runner's toenail"), which is even more common among long distance runners. It can take up to nine months for the black toenail to grow out.

SHIN PAIN

Often referred to as "shin splints," this is a pain along the shin bone, which can result from an injury to either the soft tissue or bone. Whether or not this is

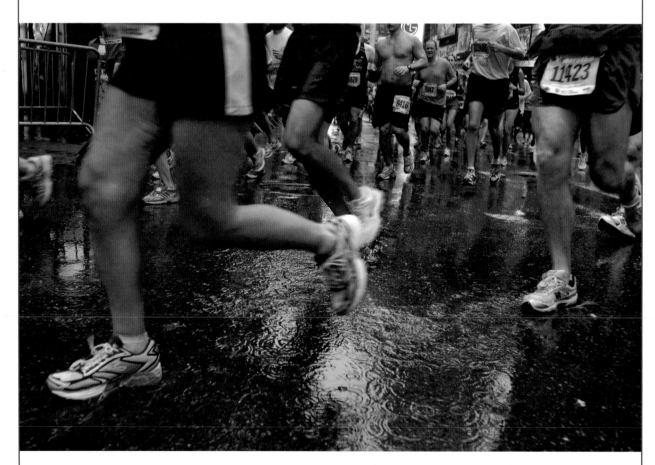

Take the necessary precautions. Rain, splashing at water stations, poorly fitting shoes or socks—any number of factors can contribute to disabling blisters.

tendinitis has to be determined by a medical professional. If it is, it will usually subside with massage, NSAIDS (anti-inflammatory medication), and a break from running. Shin splints can be caused by a variety of factors, including weaknesses of the tibialis anterior muscle, poor running biomechanics, and/or overtraining. If left untreated, it can progress to its most serious stage, a stress fracture, which is a hairline crack in the tibia or fibula, the bones of the lower leg. Rehabilitation of shin splints includes extensive rest, shoe supports, correction of errors in form, and/or stretching of the tightened calf muscles.

KNEE PAIN

Knees are undoubtedly one of the most common areas for all running injuries. In addition to bone, there are also various tendons, coming off the quadriceps muscle, that run alongside the knee. If you feel pain anywhere in or around the knee at the onset of running or walking, it is a sign to get it diagnosed. With repeated trauma, the condition will only worsen.

Chondromalacia is wear or softening of the kneecap cartilage. It can be provoked with or without running. (As we get older, bearing weight on the knee joint can create this condition). The impact of running and/or overtraining can exacerbate this problem. It is usually diagnosed by pain on resistance (a doctor will place a hand just below the knee and ask the patient to push. If this duplicates the pain, it may be chondromalacia.).

The iliotibial band (ITB) runs alongside the thigh, around the lower thigh and upper leg, and inserts around the side of the knee. Pain along the outside of the knee is most often inflammation of the ITB. It is typically felt not at the beginning of a run, but after ten or even twenty minutes. The prescription is almost always an ITB stretching program.

If you feel pain when palpating along the head (upper extremity) of the fibula, or calf bone, this may be tendinitis. It requires deep tissue massage and stretching.

BACK PAIN

Because they are close to each other anatomically, problems with the back and hip regions can result in misdiagnosis. Often there is a diagnosis of a herniated disc, when it is really inflamed soft tissue. Sometimes, the patient will submit to steroid injections and removal of a disc, resulting in long post-operative pain and recovery. Pain in the buttocks is often attributed to back problems and can even lead to the removal of a disc, when the source may actually be a soft tissue problem—tendinitis of the gluteus medius. It is caused by overuse and/or lack of flexibility. Stretching, flexibility, and deep tissue massage can be good preventive measures against further deterioration. (This can also be helpful for ITB syndrome.) When there is back pain that doesn't improve with rest and stretching, a visit to an orthopedic doctor and physical therapist can work wonders.

On the other hand, it is possible that the onset of knee pain may, in fact, originate with the lumbar spine. There may be some prolapse, or degenerative changes, in the vertebrae, particularly in the lumbosacral (lower back) region of the spine. Disc pain can also be associated with severe pain extending down the back of the thigh and leg.

Pain that originates in the upper portion of the leg and extends sometimes as far as from the butt to the feet is referred to as sciatica. It also usually originates in the back, due to pressure from the spine on the lumbar nerves. Sciatica requires a diagnosis from a medical professional. Any new onset of back pain clearly needs to be evaluated by a medical professional.

HEADACHES AND GENERAL ILLNESS

If a headache comes on while exercising, stop and see if it goes away. A persistent headache, however, needs to be medically evaluated, as there may be an underlying cause. Headaches, in addition to muscle cramps, may be a sigh of dehydration. This is particularly the case for new runners, or those who may not be acclimatized to hot or humid weather. Illness is another indication of a need to rest. If you feel sick, take a break. Don't continue to stress a sick system. A fever always indicates the need to rest. Besides, with either a bad cold or flu, no one feels like exercising anyway.

12

Marathon Nutrition and Hydration

Nutrition and hydration are crucial aspects of your marathon program. They can make all the difference for a successful outcome.

After authoring nearly a dozen books, the majority of them on running and fitness, you would think my co-author Gloria would understand everything there is to know about the marathon. But sometimes the routine closest to us—our own—can prove how little we really understand.

Gloria had run several marathons, the first dating back to what she calls "the stone age," the early 1970s. Each time, she learned from an unsuccessful experience how little she understood the event. The first time, she was undertrained. The next couple of times, which were spread out over the years, weather extremes (cold and wind, and uncharacteristic heat) should have warned her to more carefully adjust her pace. Although she regularly ran other races over the years, she understandably got fed up with the marathon.

It took her twelve years to try again, but she vowed to finally get it right. So she asked me to coach her. She promised to strictly follow the guidelines, the same ones I have given you in this book: train sensibly and use the hard/easy system (and as I have cautioned you, be as strict about the rest as the training). Even with all of this, and the advancements that had been made over the years, it was with great dismay that she reported to me after one of her first long runs that she felt the same fatigue and lightheadedness that had plagued her in past marathons.

I sensed the same problem I have seen with many runners before. An early morning runner, Gloria was used to getting by on just a cup of coffee and juice before her workout. This may support a person for a shorter run, but you can't get away with it for a longer run. I questioned her about the nutrition she had taken in for that long run (before, during, and after). I could see immediately that she had to eat more and time her intake more carefully. So from pre-run to post-run—from raisins to pancakes, sports drinks and gels—this was the beginning of a new routine based on modern sports nutrition, which has totally altered the face of marathoning. It did that for Gloria, whose "new" marathon experience (a personal best at the distance in New York at age 46 and a high placing in her age group) was revolutionized by our latest understanding of what fuels us for the long run.

Gloria wasn't alone. Once upon a time, marathoners made do merely with water, or maybe some flat soda, at best. How times have changed! No one understands this better than our friend and best-selling sports nutrition author Nancy Clark, M.S., R.D. In fact, she's written an entire book about it. Much of the advice in this chapter can be found in greater detail in that book, *Nancy Clark's Food Guide for Marathoners* (www.nancyclarkrd.com; Meyer & Meyer Sport).

GENERAL DIET

Committing to the marathon is a good way to examine, and perhaps to overhaul, your lifestyle; this includes what you eat. I feel fortunate to have been raised in Norway, where a healthy, well-balanced diet is part of our lifestyle. In fact, for my entire career, I never changed what I ate, because what worked well for my lifestyle worked well for marathon running.

Norwegians have access to an abundance of fresh foods. I take advantage of a variety of fruits and vegetables, and inexpensive whole grain bread is baked fresh daily. Our most popular cheeses, and my favorites—Gjetost and Jarlsberg—are even sold in the Unites States.

Norwegians eat a lot of fish. It is plentiful and isn't nearly as expensive as in the U.S. I eat fish at least once, sometimes twice, a day, for lunch and dinner.

In keeping with the marathon theme of good and thoughtful planning, don't get caught having to rely on poor food choices. Being a traveler has taught me by necessity to always have something healthful to eat packed in my bag. You can carry permanent non-perishables (like whole grain crackers or nuts) everywhere you go. Also, pack fruit or a sandwich if you think you may need them.

DAILY DIET

Breakfast

Nancy Clark believes that breakfast is the most important meal of the day for marathoners. Even if you're used to skipping the morning meal, she feels that you should give it a try during your marathon training, because it contributes to giving you more energy and thus stronger workouts. During my entire career, and even now, breakfast and my morning workout go together. I enjoy cooked

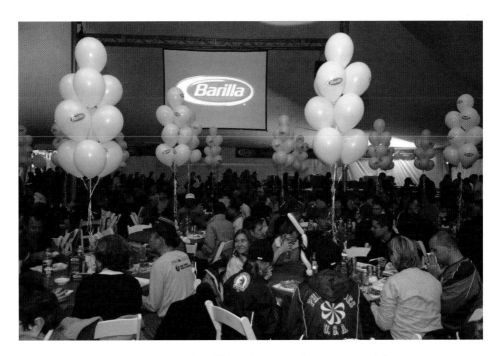

A pre-marathon pasta party. Take advantage of every aspect of the race.

cereal (oatmeal), or muesli (raw oats, dried fruits, and nuts). Muesli is common in Norway and available in the States, or you can make your own. If you don't like to cook breakfast (including French toast or pancakes), enjoy whole grain cold cereals. And if you're in a rush, make a grab-and-go peanut butter sandwich and a banana. If you like porridge, you can try what Jack and I enjoy, which is typically European. Every evening we mix our favorite dried cereal with yogurt or milk and put this in the refrigerator. In the morning, we have a healthy and satisfying porridge. And if you put it in a plastic container, it's good to go on the road.

Lunch

My lunches are very simple—baked potatoes or yams with cottage cheese, or, when I'm away from home, a Norwegian institution called a matpakke, on open-faced sandwich on thick-sliced bread. The emphasis is on the bread, with a smaller amount of protein (fish, turkey, cheese, or hard-boiled eggs). It is topped it with vegetables, such as tomatoes, cucumbers, lettuce, or cooked beets. When creating a matpakke, use your imagination; you can also try grilled vegetables or tofu. A matpakke is portable. Norway is famous for its "brown bag" habit. Even the wealthiest business people in our country bring sandwiches to work.

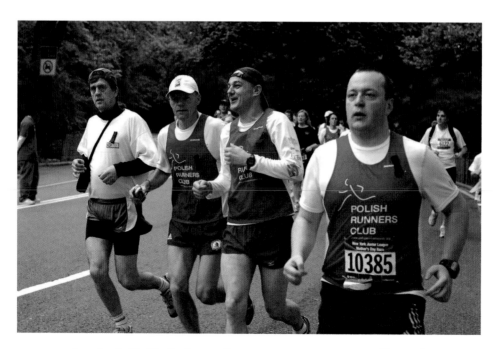

Learning to "fuel for the long run" ensures you can stay strong and focused.

Dinner

Fish is on the menu most evenings. Whatever you choose, it doesn't have to be complicated to prepare. Believe me, I'm not a cook, so I purchase as much ready-made as possible (such as sauce for fish). I combine the main course with rice or potato and a vegetable or salad. Sometimes we have chicken, or Jack likes a lean steak, but unlike in the States, chicken is more expensive than fish.

Keeping my diet very simple has always been helpful for me. As with my training, I like the routine. You can certainly choose a diet with much more variety than mine, but the important thing is to most efficiently time your eating. During my running career, I always ate three meals, supplemented with snacks, just as I do now. But I stayed away from eating heavily at one meal, or overeating in the evening. The optimal goal is to distribute your calories evenly throughout the day. This is one of the main features of Nancy Clark's advice, particularly for those who are watching their weight. If you space your eating, you'll have more energy for training (this is scientifically demonstrated in studies) and be less likely to "burn fumes" (i.e., run on empty). Well-timed eating will ultimately translate into a better marathon performance and better weight maintenance by preventing binge eating at night.

A good sports diet is comprised of all the basic food groups. It provides carbohydrates and fats to fuel the muscles, proteins to build and repair the muscles, and vitamins and minerals to regulate body functions.

What is often preached about a balanced diet especially applies during your marathon training. Now is not the time for fad diets—especially the popular non-carbohydrate or low-calorie deprivation diets. To fuel your training and provide a healthful balance, you need a variety of foods each day (fruits and vegetables, whole grains, lean meats and protein-rich foods, and low-fat milk products). Make sure to choose from at least three categories of food per meal (e.g., fish, rice, and broccoli), and two types of food groups for snacks (e.g., banana and peanut butter).

According to the American College of Sports Medicine, the best diet balance is composed of 55 to 58 percent carbohydrates; 12 to 15 percent protein; 25 to 30 percent fats.

THE MYTH ABOUT CARBOHYDRATES

Contrary to popular belief, carbohydrates are not inherently fattening. Excess calories are fattening. Wholesome carbohydrates, such as fruits, vegetables, and whole grains, should be the foundation of your sports diet. In addition, including starches, such as pasta, rice, or potatoes, is part of "carbo loading": that is, fueling your muscles to make sure you can train at your best. Nancy Clark maintains that you can also enjoy refined carbohydrates, such as sugar and soda, if desired, in moderation.

THIS IS NO TIME TO DIET

Not dieting doesn't mean you can't, or won't, lose weight during your marathon training. But Clark believes you should stop thinking about going on a diet, and start learning to eat healthfully. If you follow a sensible eating plan, you may find weight loss happens automatically. (If it doesn't, perhaps you weigh exactly what you are meant to weigh.) If you are still intent on losing weight, take Clark's advice: Don't deprive yourself; simply eat a little less (you can reasonably cut up to about 20 percent of your calories). Eat more at breakfast and lunch, so you can go "lite at night." Include a little healthful fat (e.g., avocado, nuts, olive oil) at each meal, so you don't go hungry. Finally, in keeping with the theme of your personal self-discovery through the marathon journey, learn to honor your genetics—the body you were born with—and to be realistic about your weight goals.

THERE IS NO NEED TO BE EXCESSIVELY STRICT

Clark points out that you need not have a "perfect diet" to have a good diet. While you don't want to skip a meal and fill up on sweets, 10 percent of your daily caloric intake can come from refined sugar (the amount in three small cookies or a cup of regular ice cream), and 25 percent can come from fat. Of course, try to make those healthful fats—such as olive or canola oil—but Clark's plan allows for enjoying a few high-fat treats. When I was training, I used to enjoy an afternoon indulgence of a few caramel candies or an ice cream bar. I looked forward to the ritual and saw it as a reward for doing my workouts. And I never felt guilty about it.

RUNNING DIET

A pre-exercise meal serves several functions: it staves off hunger, fuels the muscles by providing an energy boost, and helps prevent low blood sugar (thus fatigue, light headedness, or inability to focus).

Clark recommends that all marathoners practice both eating and running, since it is through trial and error that you can test what nutritional regimen works best for you. And whatever you consume, your body can also practice digesting it. While you don't want to have to digest a big meal, you don't have to starve yourself before a run. When training at a pace you can comfortably sustain, the blood flow to your stomach is 60 to 70 percent of normal, which is sufficient to maintain digestion.

However, do make sure to allow enough time between eating and running (the larger or heavier the meal, the longer digestion takes, up to three or four hours for such a meal), and experiment with liquid meals (e.g., smoothies) and small, easily digestible snacks closer to your workout.

During Your Run

In addition to hydration, for your longer runs you should ingest what you can best tolerate for quick energy (from dried fruit or candy to sports bars or gels taken with water). You will likely feel a distinct difference in your training when you consume some high-energy foods mid-run.

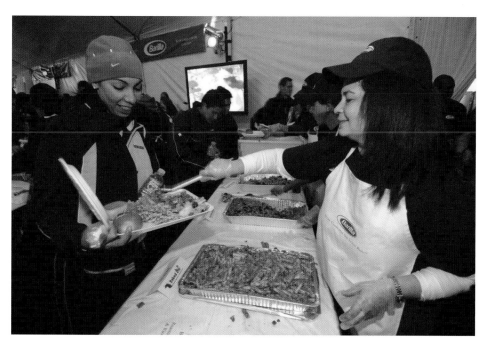

The traditional pre-race pasta meal. Runners are notorious for enjoying their food!

After Your Run

You may find you are not immediately hungry after exercise, but you should at least have a carbohydrate-based snack—such as fruit, or, better yet, a fruit and yogurt smoothie, which contains both carbs and a little protein—within 30 minutes to most efficiently refuel the muscles. You can eat a larger meal when your appetite returns.

For both training and racing, you need to practice and plan ahead. If you are scheduled for a long run, plan a course to include water stops—such as water fountains—or stash drink bottles and desired snacks or performance foods along your route. On race day, make sure you know what fluids (or performance products, like gels) are provided, and at what mile points. Better yet, break in a pair of shorts in training that include pockets for you to carry your own stash of tried and true products.

FLUIDS

During your long training runs and in the marathon, the primary goal is to prevent dehydration. Be sure to drink every fifteen to twenty minutes during exercise, or at roughly every other mile in the marathon. Drinking four to eight gulps of fluid equals the target of about four to eight ounces. Remember to drink at least that amount before and after your run as well.

You can determine more scientifically how much to drink by measuring your sweat rate. Weigh yourself before and after a one-hour run. Losing one pound in an hour means you lost one pint (sixteen ounces) of sweat, and you should drink enough to replenish that amount from now on. That translates to consuming eight ounces every half hour. Experiment with weighing yourself in various climate conditions, to get a more specific idea of your fluid needs. You should drink enough so that you lose no more than 2 percent of your weight in any exercise session. (That means losing no more than two pounds for every 100 pounds you weigh.) Check your weight often to make sure you have not lost more than 2 percent. More than that is a sign you are dehydrated.

WHAT TO DRINK

Although water (and 100 to 200 calories of a pre-exercise snack) is fine for running or walking less than an hour (and you should drink at least water during those shorter workouts), sports drinks are a helpful addition for any workout longer than that. You don't need to rely solely on a sports drink—a water/sports drink combination is most common, and gels or sports bars with water are another option. You should experiment during training with a variety of fluids to see what settles best in your stomach and what provides adequate fluids. Sports drinks also provide carbohydrates and sodium.

HYPONATREMIA—OVER HYDRATION

In the decades-long battle to fight dehydration in long distance runners, the opposite problem, overdrinking, has received wide publicity in the last several years. Overdrinking can dilute the amount of sodium (a part of salt) in your blood and lead to hyponatremia—low blood sodium. Hyponatremia can lead to nausea, fatigue, vomiting, and disorientation. In extreme cases, it can result in death. Hyponatremia can particularly become a problem for those exercising more than four hours. Beginners especially tend to drink too much, stopping at every aid station in a race, for example. You should not drink more than the recommended amount. And although sports drinks provide sodium, which helps hold water in the cells, even the standard sports drink does not offer enough sodium to prevent the possibility of hyponatremia. Most marathoners get enough sodium in their diets, even without additional salt. But especially if you are a heavy sweater, or if you run on a particularly warm day, or marathon day turns out to be a warm one, you might need some extra sodium. In this case, unless you've been advised by your doctor to avoid sodium, add salty foods to your diet (especially before and after a training run or race in which you've sweat a lot). Take some pretzels or even a small salt packet with you. If you are sweating heavily, consume either the pretzels or the salt during the later part of your long run or race.

EATING AND DRINKING TO RACE

I never changed my usual diet leading up to a race. However, I did avoid a big meal the night before a marathon, because I tended to develop stomach problems and diarrhea. I ate a bigger lunch and then had something light in the evening. Nancy Clark reports that diarrhea is common for novice runners. Their intestinal tracks may not be completely used to the marathon effort, particularly the jostling of running. (Even though I was used to it, I still had trouble.) If you fear this could be a problem for you, or if you have experienced this problem during training, experiment with your diet. Cut back on fiber and/or milk, or try lactose-free milk. If dietary changes don't work, make sure to wait at least several hours between a meal and training. Marathon courses usually feature portable toilets, but I could never afford to stop for one, which would have meant losing the race. Besides, it's no fun to have to focus on finding a toilet, especially when you don't know where they are (remember: study the race before you run, including the location of the toilets along the course). That's why I resorted to over-the-counter anti-diarrhea medications, which I took before the race. Again, regardless of what you decide to try, test it first in training.

Time of day was the biggest adjustment I had to make when I first started running the marathon, which was held in the morning. For ten years, I had run on the track, where the races are almost always in the evening. When I began running the marathon, I learned to get up very early before the race in order to have enough time to eat breakfast and allow the food to digest. I might have stocked up by increasing my food intake over the last two days, but I never overate the evening before or the morning of the race. A lot of people make that mistake. They're afraid they'll run "on empty" if they don't eat a lot. But there's only so much your body can store. Besides, you can't eat yourself to good results. It's just like training: by the time you get to the race, everything is already "in the bank." You have to eat sensibly pre-race, with the understanding that everything you put in your mouth has to be processed by your system, without disturbing your running.

The first time I ran a marathon, I did it on empty. I didn't have a sports drink. That was probably one of the key factors that made the effort so difficult. Also, trying to drink water out of paper cups while I was running wasn't easy, especially without any practice. Most of it ended up on the ground. In later years, elite runners had their own drink bottles. I timed my drinking to mimic the same procedure used in international races, which provide drinks every 5 kilometers, or three miles (the same fifteen to twenty minutes recommended for all runners). In the early part of the race, my sports drink was weaker (you can take less, or dilute it with water). Then, the solution got stronger in the later stages, as I needed more energy. I highly recommend taking gel, or some type of nutrition, particularly at about sixteen or seventeen miles. Slower marathoners should target taking in 120 to 240 carbohydrate-calories per hour of running after the first hour (the first hour is fueled by the pre-event meal).

Carry along a fanny pack. Learn to run with any nutrition or supplies you'll want in the marathon (right).

AFTER THE RACE

In my experience, most runners prepare well for the race, but as soon as they cross the finish line, they forget about recovery. The same nutrition plan you used to get to the starting line should be what you follow to recover. Make sure to have something to eat and drink as soon as you can. It seemed I hadn't

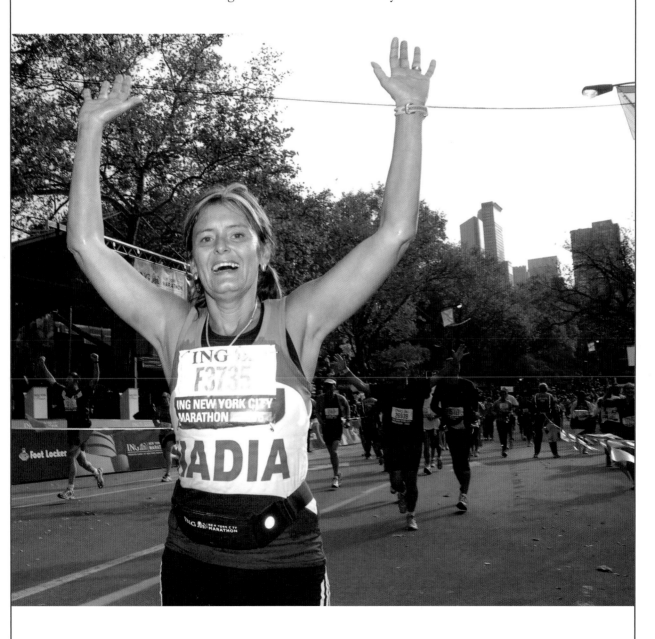

even taken my shoes off when Jack was stuffing a banana in my face. He carried a bagel in his backpack. "Eat this," he would command. I wasn't really hungry, but I knew I needed it. The sooner you eat, the sooner you recover. Most people are not hungry when they finish, so they let it go. When they get around to eating, they are overly hungry and often eat too much, too quickly. I'm amused at some marathoners' post-race habits. After the last marathon my brothers and sister-in-law ran, I found them in the hotel bar, still in their running clothes. They were drinking beer and schnapps. I wouldn't necessarily recommend it, but believe it or not, they weren't alone. There were a number of other marathoners there as well. Like my family, they were all so happy, they were celebrating.

13

The Race

The time has finally come. You've emerged from the preparation phase. Now is the time to get ready for the big day. Emerging is a good word, since, like the butterfly, becoming a marathoner is the chance to spread your wings.

TAPERING AND PEAKING

These are concepts with which runners and other athletes are very familiar. The days leading up to the race are the time for the crucial tapering and peaking. The taper, or winding down, is built into the last two weeks of your training program. This is why that time period features lower mileage, without long or strenuous running. My own taper was always two weeks. I knew that when I had done my last long run, I was basically finished. After weeks of

141

escalating training, it may seem strange to experience this decline, but as I always tell runners who feel odd or anxious at this stage, all your work is done. In the last two weeks, the training won't make you a better runner. In fact, too much running at that stage can undermine your effort. You have trained hard for fourteen weeks, and now your body needs to fully absorb that work and prepare itself for the ultimate physical and mental challenge ahead of you. Tapering doesn't mean you'll simply sit on the couch though. You'll do some running, but not as much. Some runners are very reluctant to taper because they are afraid they will lose their fitness. But you're not going to stop running; you'll simply be maintaining everything you've built up.

When you taper, you'll feel rested and have more energy. During this last two weeks, you'll also automatically become more mentally focused on the race. That's because the training is less purposeful, and that allows a necessary mental rest as well. The closer you get, the more the upcoming marathon will automatically come to mind. This was always my experience. I could feel myself gearing up. Tapering can pose a risk though, because it means you'll have more time on your hands. You may feel on edge without your usual routine. Remember, this is *not* the time to start worrying or doubting yourself (or to occupy your time by doing other heavy physical activity, like intense yard work or house cleaning, which can be draining). It's the time to think positive thoughts and to look forward to the reward for your hard work.

You taper in order to peak—to be optimally ready for the race. You rest because you want to have your best possible performance, but you can't do that for every race. In my career, peaking was for big races, like the marathon. I didn't do it for my local 10K. Ideally, you have run two other races in your training schedule, but you can't peak for every race. If you study the careers of most runners, you realize they don't run their best times in every race. It is important to understand how special, and significant, the peak is. While you can't control everything on race day, this rare peak allows you to lay the foundation for optimal success.

If a radical change in physical activity makes you feel anxious, you can continue to be physically active. Just make sure that activity is moderate. You can go for a hike, a light swim, an easy bike ride—something relaxing that still gets you moving.

In the final countdown to the race, all of the sensible lifestyle measures apply. This seems like common sense, but you'd be surprised how many people do something foolish leading up to their marathon: spring cleaning, sightseeing, or working long hours. You should minimize stress, eat well, and get enough sleep, particularly the last days before the marathon. Nerves, excitement, and a general distrust of alarm clocks might mean you don't sleep well the night before the marathon. If you do, that's great, but in my career, I never did. I always woke up several times a night. I had the classic dreams—actually, nightmares. I dreamed I was trying to follow the blue line along the New York City Marathon course, and it would run through houses and into buildings. I would be stuck in an elevator, pleading with people, "I'm supposed to be running the race!" A lot of runners tell me about their odd pre-race dreams.

I don't want to create your reality; maybe you'll sleep fine and dream of yourself flying effortlessly across the finish line. But if you do toss and turn, don't be concerned. You'll survive it for one night and still be able to run the race. It's all part of being initiated into the "marathon society."

If you're overly focused on the race and that makes you anxious, try some entertaining distractions. You suddenly have spare time when you're tapering. You can't just lie in bed, yet you don't want to tire your legs with a walk (which is why you should save any sightseeing for after the race). Often, a day or two before a big marathon, I liked to go to the movies to keep myself occupied and to forget about the race for a while. I enjoy movies; I liked being distracted and watching something that had nothing to do with running. On the other hand, some people like to revel in running. If you're new to the sport, you might get psyched up by watching some of the classic running films, such as *Chariots of Fire,* or one of the two films about Steve Prefontaine.

No matter how well prepared you are, you may experience last-minute doubts. Before most big marathons, especially as the race got closer, I went through times when I questioned myself: "Why are you doing this?" I could get very moody, even throwing my training gear all over the house, relieved that I was soon to become an ex-marathoner. Of course, the next morning I was up early for my run. Such erratic behavior is a perfectly natural response to your emotions (or so I told myself, anyway!).

GET READY…

Speaking of anxiety, people used to ask me all the time if after all my years of running, I still got nervous before a big race. Of course I did. That nervousness is a sign of "race readiness." Nerves can be good, if they are under control. Negative nervousness, the kind that wears you down with worry, can be tiring. But nervous excitement is the kind that signals you're ready and gets you psyched up!

Your anticipation can cause you to become distracted, so make sure you are well prepared. The night before the race, pack your bag, and set out your running outfit. (Some runners have their own ritual. Gloria put her gear on a chair by her bed, with her bib number pinned to her shirt, so it was the last thing she saw before she fell asleep and the first thing she saw when she woke up.) In your bag, include any old clothing you might want to wear to stay warm up until just before the start and which you're willing to discard, since you will have checked your bag beforehand. Also, add any other necessities (water, snacks, Band-Aids, petroleum jelly, etc.), especially if you're not sure what the organizers provide and if you'll be at the start a long time. If you trained with a heart rate monitor, you'll want to wear it in the race. So make sure that it's packed as well. Keep your bag with you at all times until you check it, as loss and even theft are not uncommon at crowded race starts.

If chafing is a concern, apply petroleum jelly as a preventative before you start. Don't forget sunscreen, as you can get burned on even overcast days. If you want to stay warm until you're well into the run, start with a long sleeved

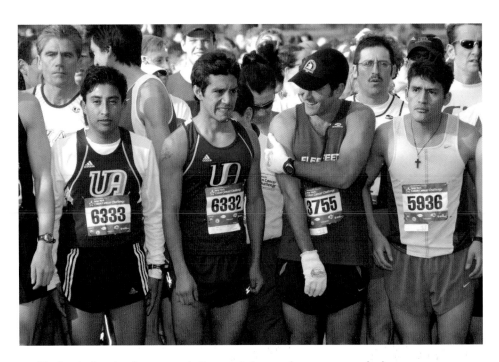

The key to dressing for success in the race is to wear layers you can shed as you warm up. Bring old clothing you can discard, or tie around your waist.

shirt over your T-shirt or singlet. Although I never ran in temperatures colder than the forties, if necessary, I used to wear a sleeveless shirt and long socks on my arms, so that I could easily pull them off when I warmed up. If the weather is quite warm, you'll have to be very careful, keeping in mind that the temperatures will likely rise even higher during your run.

Depending on the size and logistics of the race, arrive anywhere from one to four hours before the start (in mass races like New York, you don't have a choice. You have to be there several hours before. But there is plenty of food, entertainment, and group stretching sessions). Have a light breakfast at least a couple of hours before the start. Bring a bagel or banana if you're leaving very early, or if there won't be food at the start. Whatever you eat, it is just to stave off hunger, since the energy you actually run on will come mostly from the food you've had in the previous day or two.

As soon as you arrive, you'll be excited. Try to take it easy though, and conserve your energy. Find a spot to sit and relax. In my experience, the other runners around me varied in the way they liked to pass the waiting time. Some were very talkative; they liked to chat with everyone. Some listened to music. I was the type who liked to sit by myself. I just needed quiet. I used the time to think about the race, which was part of my preparation. Eventually, you might want to do a little walking and stretching, just to loosen up.

You may be nervous and begin to perspire. You'll likely need to urinate, a lot. So while you don't want to drink too much before you begin running, sipping some water before the start is a good compromise. Just make sure you scope out the toilets well before the start of the race, as there can be significantly long lines. Once you begin to run, your need to urinate should subside, particularly when you are losing fluids through sweat.

GET SET ...

When it comes time to head to the start, make sure you line up properly. In large races, get moving when you hear the first announcements. Don't wait and risk finding yourself in a panic to get situated in the proper place. There are usually large pace signs at the start to guide you, or even blocked off areas you enter according to your running number. If you are lining up on your own, be honest about where you belong. If you're too far forward, you not only risk getting trampled, you're an unfair impediment to your fellow runners. On the other hand, unless you're walking right from the start, don't position yourself all the way in the back.

While pacing is of the utmost importance, I never ran with a watch. In fact, the only time I used a watch when I ran was for intervals (timed segments in training). I taught myself to know my pace without having a watch. This comes from experience. But I also listened to my body and my inner voice. You can do this as well.

I know how unpredictable the marathon can be. That's why except for one time in my career, the Boston Marathon, I never set out to run for time, or to break a world record. Of course, my goal was to run well, and hopefully to win—but not with a clock on my mind. I paid attention to my pace, but focusing on the clock often distracts from your ability to concentrate on how your body is feeling. And in this race, that can be fatal.

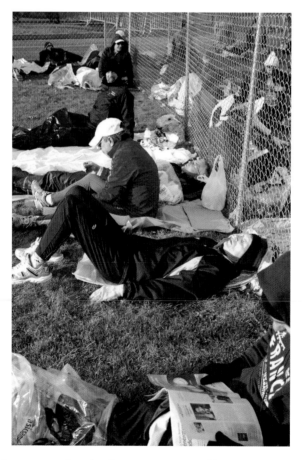

Chat, rest, meditate—stay relaxed and save your energy while waiting at the marathon start.

Be flexible. You may have to make adjustments to your marathon plan. If the weather is hot or humid, it is even more important to run conservatively, recognizing it will add minutes to your finishing time. If you are ill, especially if you have a fever, or you're injured, you should not attempt to run. You'll be much safer and guarantee a better experience if you allow yourself to recover and save your training effort for a race you can successfully complete.

GO!

The start: It's everything you've trained toward and waited for. It's exciting, all right—but also potentially risky. You are rested and motivated, and that is

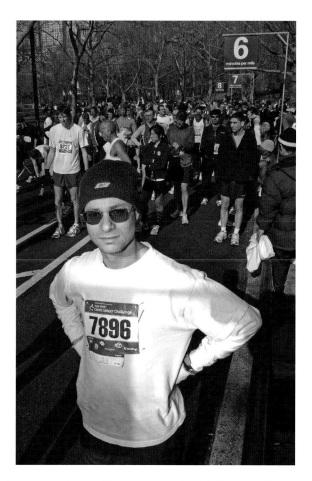

Large pace signs guide runners on where to line up at the start.

what will allow you to get through 26.2 miles. But it will also make you prone to the sin of inexperience: being pulled out too fast by the pack, the crowds, and your own adrenaline. If there are a lot of runners, it may be slow going to get over the starting line. However, major marathons now feature shoe chip technology, which also records your time based on when you cross the rubber mat at the starting line. Even so, the first mile or even two can be congested. Try to see it as a blessing; it can keep you from running too quickly. Don't panic. You have plenty of miles to make up the time.

Make sure to get into the same rhythm you used for your long training runs. You'll want the same pace as those twenty-milers. If you've trained with walking breaks, make sure to use them in the race. Remind yourself to stay calm. Nervousness can cause rapid or shallow breathing and consequently cramps or stitches.

When you're caught up in the anticipation and excitement of the start, it's easy to make the most common mistake during the race—to think only in the moment, instead of about the hours ahead. In terms of my mentality, I always ran thinking about the last six miles. When I got to that point, I wanted to feel I could increase the pace. I think that's why I never truly "hit the wall" in a marathon. I ran negative splits (the second half quicker than the first) or at an even pace. As I came to the last three or four miles—the tough part for nearly everyone—I'd build my confidence by thinking of familiar distances back home, telling myself, "This is to the store and back." It was comforting to focus on a course I'd run often, without problems.

It will probably take you a few miles to get fully into your rhythm. You may feel quite good for quite a while and thoroughly enjoy the race. That's great. Look around; soak in the atmosphere. Eventually, however, you will reach the point where you may be feeling something you haven't experienced in training. It's a different type of fatigue and muscle soreness, caused by the pounding. You feel it mostly in the quadriceps (front of your thighs). This is why the walking breaks are a good idea. My sister-in-law Wenche, who used walking, never felt that soreness. However, although you may not experience problems, even Wenche had to grit her teeth with about four miles to go. That's the final push home, and it takes effort. You may have to postpone your sense of enjoyment until it's over and you've crossed the finish line. Of course, I've talked to first-time marathoners who had no problems at all. They tell me they could have run faster.

The final miles are where positive thinking comes in. At that point, you know you're getting close to the finish line; you're determined to get there. Just start talking to yourself. Tell yourself, "One leg after the other; I'll be there soon; keep on going." I talked to myself often in a marathon, "Only four miles; that's my neighborhood loop; I can do that."

Sometimes, you have your day. You run great, and you just can't explain it. In several of my marathons, the last several miles felt like I was flying. I wish I had some magic formula to share, but the truth is I ran only three marathons where everything clicked. You can only try your best to get it right. There are factors you can't control. Most of my races had their tough patches. But that's the beauty of it; making it to the finish line despite the challenges.

PACING

Pacing yourself during the race deserves its own section, since it is the number one factor in determining your marathon experience. In order to get your

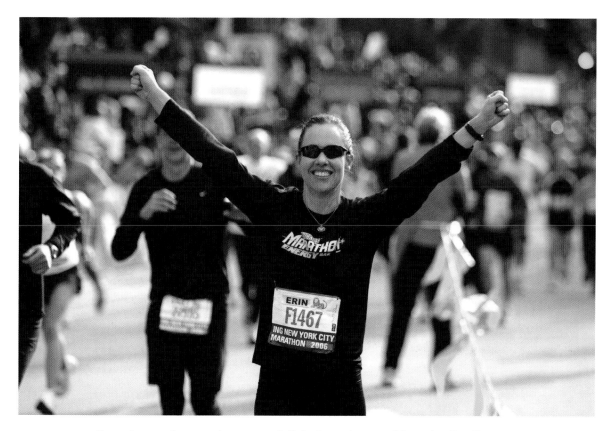

Savor the marathon experience, especially in the excitement of the early miles. However, also keep your attention focused on your effort.

pacing right, you must hold back in the early stages to make sure you can get to the finish line. Trust me, even if you feel great the first five miles—you're all pumped, your legs are light—that's not going to last. That's why, while you enjoy the moment, you have to be vigilant about what lies ahead of you.

Proper pacing takes great discipline. I told Wenche to take it easy and to jog/walk from the beginning. She stuck with the program religiously. But my brothers, who were running with her, were trying to push her along. She was angry. She knew she had to stay on pace. She was getting tired and didn't like being pushed. "I almost divorced him out there," she joked to me about my brother Arild.

So many runners I meet are afraid of "hitting the wall." I assure them that if they are prepared and pace themselves properly, there is no law that says they're going to hit the wall. But the fear of the wall is so notorious that some runners assume it's inevitable. "What will happen when I hit the wall?" they ask me. I tell them if they really want to see, go out at too quick a pace and they'll surely find out.

I know I've just told you in the section above that I never hit the wall. Although I didn't recognize it at the time, that may have happened to me in my first marathon. It was caused by lack of experience, insufficient preparation, and dehydration. The last five miles I really struggled. But the fact I pushed through is proof that even if you do hit the wall, it doesn't mean it's immovable.

When you truly hit the wall, you feel you can't go on. You slow down. You have to walk. Maybe you start to jog again, but you just can't pick it up the pace. That doesn't mean you can't walk the rest of the way, depending on where you are. But that's not the way you've prepared to finish.

One of the ways to ensure proper pacing is not to do battle with your body. Both physically and mentally, avoid getting into the pushing or struggling mode. Most runners face this challenge, the temptation to put pressure on themselves. When I used to put pressure on myself to force the pace, my body would tighten up, and that would affect my form. I tended to "tie up." This happened most often during my track career, but it was a good lesson for me on the roads. Instead of going into the "panic" mode, I would tell myself to relax (you can do that physically, by focusing on dropping your shoulders or shaking out your arms). A race should be a test of ability, not survival. If you focus on that relaxation, it will help.

My husband Jack has been with me every step of the way. He's been to so many marathons and talked to so many people that he is remarkably fluent in the event. In addition to what he learned during my career, he learned personally, and the hard way. He made the most typical mistake of first timers. Over the years, he shared his resulting wisdom with me: Remember, the race isn't over until you've crossed the finish line. Never lose confidence when you go through bad patches, he also told me.

JACK WAITZ: I was aware of the reputation of the marathon, that is, it's different than other running. But you have to experience it to truly understand it. Even being around Grete in her marathon career, I

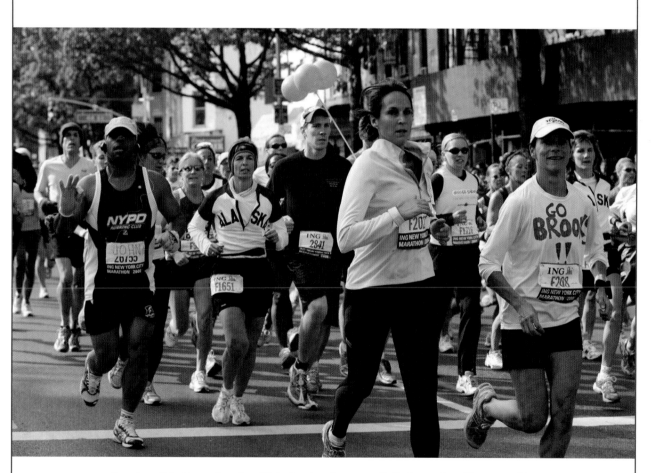

Easy does it. In the early going, think about saving yourself. Find a comfortable pace, with a like-minded pack.

didn't realize what the race is about on a personal level. You can learn from someone else, but that's very hard. It's never like going through it yourself. Still, over the years, I have told a lot of others to learn from my experience. Some do. It varies. It may be more of a male than a female thing to make the mistake I did the first time out. Women may be a little more careful.

My first marathon was in Stockholm, when I was 36. It was basically a mistake in pacing. I wasn't used to the distance. You have no respect for what is going to happen after eighteen miles. Most people are in good shape, so you go a certain distance feeling fine, and then it hits you.

I was feeling great up until the halfway. It was a piece of cake. A few miles later, it was over. My body just shut down. I had to drop out. Up until then, the pace didn't feel at all too quick. You're used to running faster, for shorter distances. Suddenly, you're in a marathon, running slower, and you think: this is easy. It's very important to pace yourself according to the distance, to find the right pace you can handle for the long run. Of course, this isn't always so easy.

Even though it was painful, and I dropped out, I was sure I wanted to try it again—to do it right. I chose to do the same race the following year. This time, I did a few more long runs in training, but the basic change was in my pacing. That made a huge difference. The margin between running the right pace and too fast can be very small (maybe just a few seconds a mile), but the result is quite dramatic. I was able to run the two halves in more or less even pace, and I finished in decent shape. It also had to do with the day. You feel different from day to day. One day you're fine; another day you have problems. I wanted to do it right this time, and to finish, so some of my effort was mental. But in the end, it all came down to that pacing. You're trained to go the distance. If you do everything else you are supposed to, the only thing that could ruin it is if you run too fast.

Over the years, I ended up running eight marathons in all. After my experience and all the years of watching Grete and other runners, I still firmly believe the most important aspect is pacing. If you have prepared the way you should and have some guidance, you'll do okay. But you probably need some help, someone to evaluate your training. I had a group of friends I ran with. We were very careful to stay together and to keep the proper pace. Some guys were more disciplined than others.

After my first marathon experience, I was very aware that I had to run a certain pace, and I tried to control the other guys in the group. That paid off for us all.

Throughout her entire marathon career, Grete had a lot of control. She did extremely well with pacing. On one hand, she may have been able to run some of her races faster, if she did them differently, but her goal wasn't time, it was to win. Running a race for time can be a big gamble. She wasn't the gambling type with a race like the marathon. Mainly, she was extremely disciplined. That's her personality. She knew what she had to do to get through the race, and she was also very smart about it.

DNF (DID NOT FINISH)

Of course, I'm an advocate for finishing what you start. Part of the discipline of running a marathon is sticking it out and seeing it through. However, you also accept that it's a gamble. It's a long race, with the potential for serious risk. Obviously, it's challenging, but there's a difference between difficulty and danger. You may experience a natural fatigue you have to endure and conquer, but that's not the same as illness or injury.

I have never dropped out of a race, except for the marathon. It happened twice, and both times, I had no choice. In one New York City Marathon I was injured, and whether or not I could push through it, it wasn't worth doing further damage. The second time, in Boston, at twenty-three miles, my body simply shut down. (I had a warning sign when my legs began to tire at fifteen miles, much too soon for that to be happening.) It's not exactly positive thinking to address this topic, and I'm certainly not suggesting you put it in the forefront of your mind. However, you do need to understand and respect safety issues. Each of us has our own pain threshold, but if you feel in doubt at any point along the way, use common sense. It's not worth risking your health or hurting yourself. If you are concerned at any point, consult the race medical personnel immediately. They are usually along the course.

If you don't make it due to injury or illness, or if your legs just can't carry you, don't be discouraged. You can do another marathon. You should give yourself some time to recover, however. Rest a couple of weeks, find another race, and resume the training schedule to include at least another few long runs. In the meantime, learn from your experience. Look back and try to discover where you went wrong. Evaluate your race. Was there anything that impacted your effort, such as dehydration or improper pacing? Look through your diary and try to determine if there were any areas in your preparation that may have caused a problem, or on which you can improve.

Sometimes, you can't explain it. In that particular race, you just didn't have a good day. You may not know what went wrong, but chalk it up to experience, knowing you can try to get it right the next time.

THE REWARD

You've finally done it. You've completed a marathon. Now is the time for celebration and reward. But before you savor your experience, be aware that your race doesn't exactly end after you've crossed the finish line. Many people make the mistake of failing to properly recover from a marathon.

Just as it is important to warm up, it is important to unwind from the race. All the steps you took to prepare in getting ready are the same ones you should follow to cool down. Once you cross the line, keep moving. Avoid the urge to sit down. (I've seen many a runner sitting on a curb who I am convinced was still there because he or she couldn't get up!) Keep walking. And keep warm. Some races have metallic-looking blankets (they are made of mylar) that are handed out to keep you warm, but it is still important to change into dry clothes as soon as you can. The cooler the temperature, the more quickly you need to do this.

Get something to drink, and take in some nutrition. Often, with the effort and excitement, you won't feel hungry. But for optimal recovery, you should eat something within thirty to sixty minutes after the event. Many runners wait too long, until they are very hungry, and then tend to overeat. If you have any physical or medical concerns, take care of them right away, including blisters (they can get infected if not properly treated). There are medical personnel at the finish.

If there is no designated spot to rendezvous with family and friends, set up a meeting place well ahead of time. Make it specific and preferably away from the crowds. You can become quite disoriented after the race, and there are many cases of those who hunted around in vain for their friends or relatives.

Eat a recovery diet, and hydrate, which is similar to how you prepared by building up for the event. Over the next few days and weeks, walk and stretch to aid recovery and always before resuming running.

Finally, how should you evaluate your experience? If you had a goal and met it, that's wonderful. You should be happy if you made it to the finish.

If you had a great time and enjoyed the run, that's even better. If you feel you could have run faster, that's a bonus too. It might motivate you to try again.

If you do want to run another marathon, use the same training program. However, if you want to improve, you will have to be more prepared. The program in the book is a basic one. Improving your time will require more running, over a longer period of time. You will likely have to increase your mileage and include a few more long runs.

You can become a regular, lifetime runner and never do another marathon. If you want to run other races, that's fine, but you can simply maintain quality fitness by running at least four to six miles, four times a week.

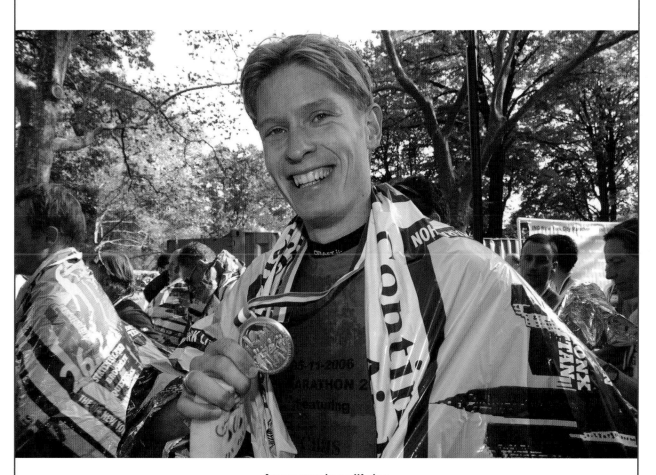

A memory to last a lifetime.

Mary Wittenberg has been with New York Road Runners for eight years and serves the organization as president and chief operating officer, as well as race director for the New York City Marathon. She won the 1987 Marine Corps Marathon in 2:44 and competed in the 1988 U.S. Olympic Marathon Trials. What impresses me about Mary is how she runs such a big organization, comes to almost every weekend race, travels all over the world, is the mother of two, and still manages to run herself. Her lifestyle takes my breath away.

MARY WITTENBERG: Finishing a marathon is a life-affirming event, and your celebration should reflect that. Race evening is a time to have fun, enjoy yourself, and relish your success. Your family and friends have probably sacrificed a lot for you, so it's a wonderful time to celebrate together with them as well.

If you immediately focus on your next goal, you miss out on the opportunity to celebrate. In the New York City Marathon, we have the evening dancing and awards ceremony. We also have 5,000 people show up at the finish line the following day beginning at 7 a.m. to celebrate with other runners. They can get their finisher's medals engraved, purchase marathon merchandise, view the race broadcast on a big-screen TV, and meet the race winners for autographs.

The day after the race is the first day in a long time you're not worried about running. This is a time to be social, as well as to feel good about yourself. So set up a schedule to walk with friends for the next days or weeks.

So many people get lured in by the power and drama of the marathon as their major goal. Once they achieve it, however, their greater goal should really be to become lifetime runners. Following their first marathon is the time of greatest risk for potential lifetime runners. Some people run the next morning (actually, you're better off walking), while some completely stop running for good.

The marathon is a great goal, whatever way you look at it, as a lifetime achievement, and it is the best platform you'll have for staying fit for life. Of course, you'll want to take it easy for the next couple of weeks, but then start jogging again. It can be hard to get out running after your recovery, especially the first session or two. But you actually have a tremendous fitness base after training for and doing the marathon. You can pick your next (shorter) race, something lower key, to run for fun. Then, you can set other goals for the future.

People don't often realize it, but there is a natural risk of feeling low, or depressed, after finishing a marathon. I think it's both psychological and physiological. It's such a big goal. It's likely on the list of major feats you want to accomplish in life, so naturally you feel a bit empty when it's over. Less glamorous, but just as important, is the lifelong fitness habit the marathon inspires. The sooner you get training after your break, the better.

RESOURCES

Road Runners Club of American (RRCA)
www.rrca.org
An organization of over 700 clubs and 180,000 members.

New York Road Runners
www.nyrr.org
The largest club of its kind in the world. They conduct the New York City Marathon and boast a full yearly calendar of events.

Association of International Marathons and Road Races (AIMS)
www.aims-association.org
An association of more than 230 race organizations located in eighty countries. AIMS' calendar of member races is made up of accredited races.

Runner's World Online
www.runnersworld.com
Everything about running. The Web site from the leading national magazine.

MarathonGuide.com
www.marathonguide.com
Everything marathon—information, results, advice and more.

Running Times Online
www.runningtimesmagazine.com
Articles and information from this long-running national magazine.

Marathon-World.com
www.marathon-world.com
A directory of links to 533 marathon races in sixty-four countries on all seven continents.

Cool Running
www.coolrunning.com
Information on every aspect of running, for every level.

LetsRun.com
www.letsrun.com
An "everything Web site" for road running and track and field. Also dedicated to improving performance.

Serpentine Running Club
www.serpentine.org.uk
Extensive advice for all levels of runners, notably from English coach Frank Horwill.

Run-Down
www.run-down.com
Links to other sites and resources.

Runner Girl
www.runnergirl.com
Expert advice for girls and women athletes of all ages and all levels.

Running Network
www.runningnetwork.com
Calendar of events, training tips, eNewsletter.

Run the Planet
www.runtheplanet.com
Running tips, races, and routes for runners worldwide.

ACKNOWLEDGMENTS

Thanks to New York Road Runners and Susan Cuttler and Jillian Haber, David Lowenthal, M.D., Ph.D., Nancy Clark M.S., R.D., John Stanton, John Fabbro, Vebjorn Rogne, Team Trykk, Paul Friedman, and Jack Waitz.

ABOUT THE AUTHORS

GRETE WAITZ

Grete Waitz, born in Norway, is arguably the most accomplished long distance runner of all time. Among her achievements, she is a nine-time New York City Marathon winner, the 1983 World Championships marathon winner, and the 1984 Olympic marathon silver medalist. She set three world records in the marathon. Prior to her marathon career, she spent a decade as an Olympian and world record holder on the track and was also a five-time World Cross Country champion. She is the author of running, health, and fitness books in English and Norwegian and has coached thousands of runners of all levels. Since her retirement from competitive running, Waitz has worked on promoting health and fitness in the United States and Europe.

GLORIA AVERBUCH

Gloria Averbuch is the author of eleven books on exercise, health, and fitness, two of them co-authored with Grete Waitz. Among them is *The New York Road Runners Club Complete Book of Running & Fitness*, which was called "the most useful and comprehensive running book ever" by *Runner's World* magazine. It is currently in its fourth edition. She is a masters runner and worked for the New York Road Runners for over twenty years.

INDEX